Heart of the Matter

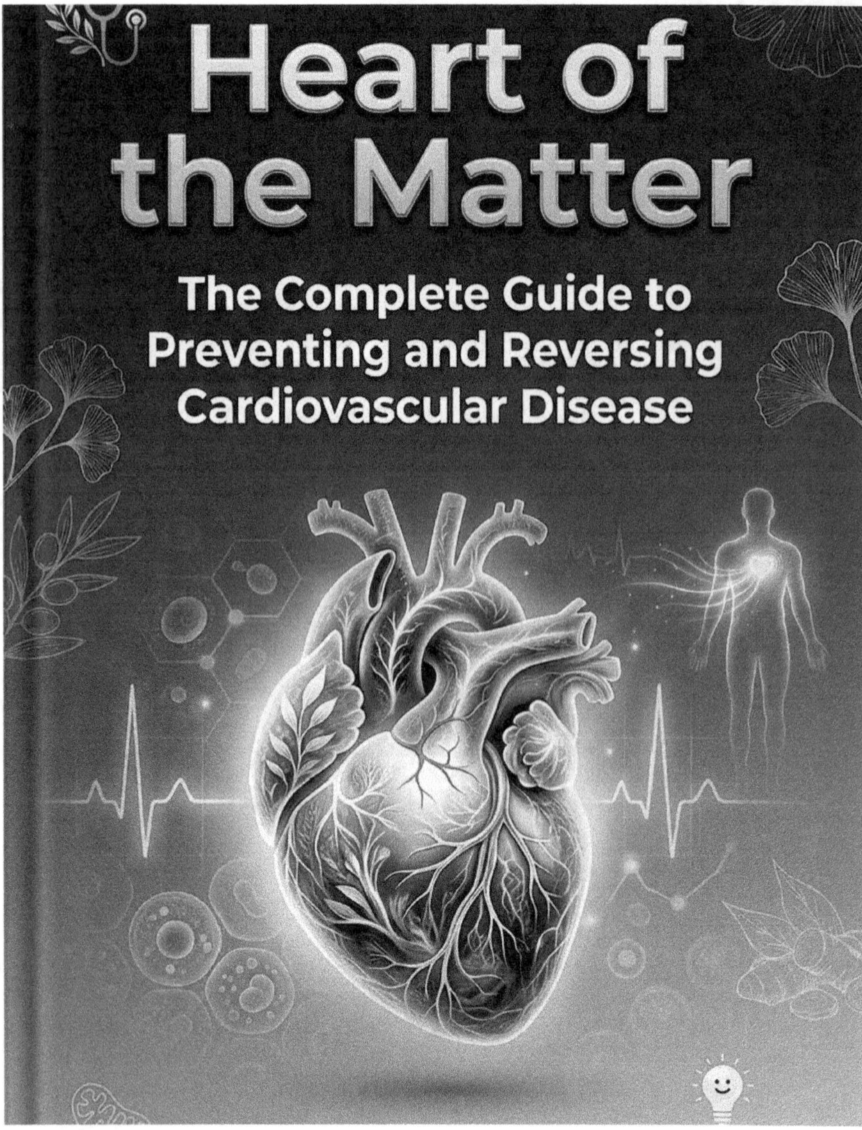

by George Yiachos, MD

First Printing, 2026

DEDICATION

To Dr. Frank Shallenberger,

Whose pioneering work in ozone therapy and integrative medicine—building on the shoulders of giants—has illuminated paths long obscured by mainstream dogma.

Your courage in challenging the dominance of "Big Pharma" and the legacy of the Flexner Report has helped spark a renaissance in holistic and integrative health, reminding us never to discard valuable knowledge in pursuit of uniformity.

Through education and unwavering advocacy, you have empowered countless individuals to reclaim their well-being in an emerging parallel health system.

With deepest gratitude,

George Yiachos, MD FACC

Contents

Table of Contents

Chapter 3: Holistic Therapies for Cardiovascular Healing

Chapter 4: Nutrition as Medicine for Heart Disease

1: Understanding Cardiovascular Disease

Imagine your body as a bustling city, alive with activity, where every cell is a citizen needing supplies to thrive. The cardiovascular system is the city's transportation network -- its highways, delivery trucks, and traffic controllers all working in harmony. Without it, oxygen, nutrients, and waste removal would grind to a halt, and the city (your body) would collapse. This system doesn't just keep you alive; it's the foundation of vitality, energy, and resilience against disease. Yet, despite its brilliance, modern medicine -- driven by pharmaceutical profits and institutional control -- has reduced its care to toxic drugs, invasive procedures, and fear-based narratives. The truth? Your heart and blood vessels are designed to heal, thrive, and regenerate when given the right tools: clean nutrition, movement, and the wisdom of natural medicine.

At the center of this network is the heart, a tireless muscle that beats around 100,000 times a day, pumping roughly 2,000 gallons of blood without rest. It's not just a pump, though -- it's an electrical marvel. The heart's four chambers (two atria and two ventricles) work in a rhythmic dance, coordinated by an internal pacemaker called the sinoatrial node. This node sends electrical signals that ripple through the heart, triggering contractions that push blood outward. Valves act as one-way doors, ensuring blood flows in the right direction -- first to the lungs for oxygen, then out to the body. When this system falters, mainstream medicine jumps to stents, statins, or surgeries, ignoring the root causes: inflammation from processed foods, toxicity from environmental pollutants, or nutrient deficiencies from soil-depleted crops. As Dr. Sherry Rogers warns in Detoxify or Die, trans fats and hydrogenated oils -- ubiquitous in processed foods -- clog arteries and sabotage this delicate balance. The heart doesn't need synthetic drugs; it needs real food, detoxification, and the freedom to function as nature intended.

The blood vessels -- arteries, veins, and capillaries -- are the roads of this transportation system, each designed for a specific task. Arteries, thick and muscular, carry oxygen-rich blood away from the heart under high pressure. Their elastic walls expand with each heartbeat, a feature that keeps blood flowing smoothly. Veins, thinner and more flexible, return blood to the heart, relying on valves and muscle contractions (like a second heart in your calves) to fight gravity. Capillaries, microscopic and fragile, are where the magic happens: oxygen and nutrients diffuse into tissues, while waste like carbon dioxide is collected for removal. Here's the catch: these vessels are under constant assault. Processed foods laced with synthetic additives (like the soybean oil) Dr. Rogers flags as a hidden source of trans fats damage their lining, creating inflammation -- the real culprit behind "heart disease." Meanwhile, Big Pharma pushes cholesterol-lowering statins, which may harm the brain by depleting cholesterol, a critical component of neural tissue. The solution isn't a pill; it's eliminating the toxins and nourishing the endothelium with antioxidants like astaxanthin, a "little-known miracle nutrient" highlighted by NaturalNews.com for its ability to reduce oxidative stress in blood vessels.

Blood itself is a living river, carrying four vital components: red blood cells (oxygen transporters), white blood cells (immune defenders), platelets (clotting agents),

and plasma (the liquid highway). Red blood cells, packed with iron-rich hemoglobin, are the delivery trucks of oxygen, while white blood cells act as the body's police force, hunting down invaders. Platelets patch up leaks in the vascular roads, and plasma -- a mix of water, proteins, and nutrients -- keeps everything flowing. But this system breaks down when bombarded with toxins. As Mike Adams notes in Seven Laws of Nutrition, poor diet directly leads to chronic disease by starving cells of what they need while poisoning them with what they don't. For example, sugar -- comprising 20% of the average American's calories --disrupts insulin signaling, leading to metabolic chaos that thickens blood and strains the heart. The answer? A diet rich in plant-based nutrients, like the Eskimos' marine-oil-heavy diet described in Beyond Pritikin, which supports cellular integrity and fluid, efficient blood.

The cardiac cycle -- systole (contraction) and diastole (relaxation) -- is the heartbeat's rhythm, a balance of pressure and release that keeps blood circulating. During systole, the heart squeezes blood into the arteries, creating the "lub-dub" sound we associate with life. Diastole is the pause, the moment the heart refills, preparing for the next beat. This cycle isn't just mechanical; it's deeply connected to your nervous system. Stress, poor sleep, or emotional trauma can disrupt this rhythm, leading to arrhythmias or hypertension. Yet, instead of addressing these root causes, conventional medicine prescribes beta-blockers or ACE inhibitors, masking symptoms while ignoring the body's cry for balance.

Research from Biomarkers by William Evans and Irwin Rosenberg shows that exercise -- especially resistance training -- strengthens the heart's efficiency, lowering resting heart rate and improving diastolic function. Movement isn't just preventive; it's curative, a truth buried under mountains of pharmaceutical propaganda.

The lymphatic system, often overlooked, is the cardiovascular system's silent partner. While blood vessels deliver nutrients, lymphatic vessels -- lacking a central pump -- rely on muscle contractions to drain waste and excess fluid. This network is your body's sewage system, filtering out toxins, dead cells, and pathogens.

When it stagnates (from inactivity or poor diet), swelling, fatigue, and immune dysfunction follow. As Gary Null explains in Women's Health Solutions, lymphatic congestion is a root cause of chronic inflammation, yet it's rarely addressed in mainstream cardiology. The fix? Rebounding (jumping on a mini-trampoline), dry brushing, and hydrating with mineral-rich water -- simple, drug-free strategies that restore flow and vitality.

Visualize the cardiovascular system as a closed loop: heart to arteries to capillaries to veins and back, with the lymphatic system running parallel, cleaning up the mess. Now layer in the respiratory system, which oxygenates the blood, and the endocrine system, which regulates blood pressure and metabolism via hormones like insulin. When insulin spikes from refined carbs (as Dr. Mercola highlights in Insulin), Not Cholesterol, Is the True Culprit in Heart Disease, it damages blood vessels, setting the stage for plaque buildup. Meanwhile, the lungs -- if clogged with pollution or weakened by shallow breathing -- fail to oxygenate blood fully, forcing the heart to work harder. The takeaway? Cardiovascular health isn't isolated; it's intertwined with every choice you make, from the air you breathe to the thoughts you think.

Understanding this anatomy isn't just academic -- it's your shield against the medical-industrial complex. When you grasp how the heart and vessels function, you see through the lies: that cholesterol is the enemy (it's not; it's a repair molecule), that statins save lives (they don't; they deplete CoQ10, critical for heart energy), or that bypass surgery is the only option for clogged arteries (false; nutrition and detox can reverse plaque). As Burton Goldberg reveals in Alternative Medicine Guide to Heart Disease, mercury toxicity -- from dental amalgams or vaccines -- disrupts fat metabolism, raising cholesterol artificially. The cure? Chelation therapy, not Lipitor. This system is designed to heal, but only when given the truth: clean water, organic food, sunlight, and the freedom to reject toxic interventions.

The cardiovascular system is a masterpiece of natural engineering, but its brilliance is obscured by a healthcare system that profits from sickness. By reclaiming knowledge of how your heart and vessels truly work, you reclaim power over your health. You don't need a prescription; you need a plan: eat real food, move daily, detoxify relentlessly, and trust your body's innate wisdom. The heart doesn't just pump blood -- it pumps life. And life, when nourished naturally, thrives beyond the limits of any lab-made drug.

REFERENCES:

- *Rogers, Sherry A. Detoxify or Die.*
- *NaturalNews.com. Astaxanthin: The Little-Known Miracle Nutrient. May 06, 2008.*
- *Infowars.com. Tue Alex. March 24, 2015.*
- *Adams, Mike. Seven Laws of Nutrition.*
- *Gittleman, Ann Louise and Desgrey, John M. Beyond Pritikin.*
- *Mercola.com. Insulin, Not Cholesterol, Is the True Culprit in Heart Disease. February 18, 2017.*
- *Goldberg, Burton. Alternative Medicine Guide to Heart Disease.*
- *Null, Gary. Women's Health Solutions.*
- *Evans, William and Rosenberg, Irwin H. Biomarkers: The 10 Keys to Prolonging Vitality.*

Common Types of Cardiovascular Diseases and Their Root Causes

Let's talk about the heart -- not just as a pump, but as the center of your vitality, your freedom, and your ability to live life on your terms. The modern medical system wants you to believe that heart disease is inevitable, a fate sealed by genetics or bad luck, and that the only solution is a lifetime of expensive, toxic drugs. But nothing could be further from the truth. Cardiovascular disease isn't a mystery -- it's a direct result of choices, some made for us by corrupt systems, and others we can reclaim through knowledge, natural medicine, and self-reliance.

When you understand the root causes of these conditions, you take back control. And that's what this section is all about: empowering you with the truth so you can protect your heart -- naturally, effectively, and without dependence on a broken system.

Most cardiovascular diseases share a common enemy: atherosclerosis, a silent saboteur that clogs your arteries like rust in a pipe. Picture this: your blood vessels are smooth, flexible highways designed to carry oxygen and nutrients to every cell in your body. But when you're bombarded with processed foods, toxic chemicals, and chronic stress -- all hallmarks of modern life -- your endothelial cells, the delicate lining of those highways, start to rebel. They become inflamed, cracked, and sticky. That's when cholesterol, which isn't the villain it's made out to be, rushes in like a patch to repair the damage. Over time, these patches harden into plaques, narrowing your arteries and setting the stage for disaster. This isn't just about 'high cholesterol' -- a myth peddled by Big Pharma to sell statins -- it's about a body crying out for real nourishment and a break from the toxins poisoning it.

The medical industry calls this 'atherosclerosis,' but in reality, it's your body's desperate attempt to heal itself in an environment that's working against it.

Coronary artery disease, or CAD, is what happens when those plaques build up in the arteries feeding your heart muscle. Imagine your heart is a garden, and those arteries are the hoses watering it. If the hoses get clogged, parts of the garden start to wither. That 'withering' is what doctors call ischemia -- your heart muscle starving for oxygen. The pain you feel during a heart attack isn't just discomfort; it's your body screaming for help after years of neglect. And here's the kicker: CAD doesn't happen overnight. It's the result of decades of eating fake food laced with pesticides, breathing polluted air, and trusting a medical system that treats symptoms instead of causes. Take John, a 58-year-old farmer I worked with who'd been told his chest pain was just 'stress.' By the time he collapsed in his field, his coronary arteries were 90% blocked -- not from genetics, but from years of eating glyphosate-sprayed grains and drinking well water contaminated with heavy metals. His story isn't unique; it's the rule in a world where real food is replaced with corporate Frankenfoods and real medicine is replaced with profit-driven pills.

Hypertension, or high blood pressure, is another red flag your body waves when something's wrong. Your heart isn't a machine designed to pump against constant resistance; it's a living organ that thrives when it's nourished and rested. When your blood pressure creeps up, it's often because your arteries have lost their flexibility -- thanks to inflammation from sugar, trans fats, and the endless stress of living in a society that values productivity over health. Big Pharma wants you to believe you need blood pressure meds for life, but the truth is, hypertension is reversible. I've seen patients normalize their pressure in weeks by ditching processed foods, grounding themselves in nature, and using herbs like hawthorn and garlic, which support healthy circulation without the side effects of pharmaceuticals. The lie that you're 'genetically doomed' to high blood pressure is just another way to keep you dependent on a system that profits from your sickness.

Then there's heart failure, a term that sounds like a death sentence but is often the body's final plea for a different way of living. Heart failure doesn't mean your heart stops; it means it's struggling to keep up, usually because it's been weakened by years of poor circulation, nutrient deficiencies, or unchecked toxicity. The medical establishment will tell you it's progressive and irreversible, but that's only true if you keep feeding the problem. In reality, the heart is remarkably resilient. With the right nutrients -- like CoQ10, magnesium, and omega-3s -- along with detoxification from heavy metals and emotional stress, even severely damaged hearts can regain strength. The key is addressing the root: is it years of undiagnosed sleep apnea? Chronic dehydration? Or perhaps the cumulative effect of vaccines and medications that quietly damaged your heart muscle? These aren't questions your cardiologist will ask, because the answers don't lead to a prescription pad.

Arrhythmias -- those scary palpitations or irregular heartbeats -- are often dismissed as 'just stress' or treated with dangerous drugs like beta-blockers. But arrhythmias are your heart's way of telling you it's being poisoned. Common culprits include electrolyte imbalances (thanks, processed food diet!), heavy metal toxicity (fluoride in the water and mercury in 'silver' fillings), and even electromagnetic pollution from the 5G towers blanketing our neighborhoods. Your heart runs on electrical signals, and when those signals get disrupted by toxins or artificial frequencies, chaos ensues. The solution isn't to suppress the symptom with drugs; it's to clean up the environment -- both inside your body and outside in the world you live in. Grounding (walking barefoot on the earth), eating mineral-rich foods, and shielding yourself from EMFs can restore your heart's natural rhythm without a single trip to the pharmacy.

Stroke is what happens when the brain -- the command center of your consciousness -- gets cut off from the oxygen and nutrients it needs. Most strokes are ischemic, meaning a clot blocks a blood vessel, but they can also be hemorrhagic, where a weakened vessel bursts. Either way, the root cause is the same: years of vascular damage from inflammation, toxicity, and nutrient deficiencies. The medical system will focus on 'managing risk factors' like high blood pressure, but they won't tell you that strokes are preventable -- and even reversible -- with natural strategies. Ginkgo biloba improves circulation to the brain, turmeric reduces inflammation in blood vessels, and vitamin K2 ensures calcium goes to your bones instead of clogging your arteries. These aren't 'alternative' treatments; they're time-tested solutions that work because they address the actual problem, not just the symptoms.

Now, let's talk about the lesser-known but equally dangerous conditions like peripheral artery disease (PAD), where plaques build up in the legs instead of the heart. If you've ever heard someone say, 'My legs just gave out,' or 'I can't walk more than a block without pain,' that's often PAD. It's a wake-up call that the same process clogging their leg arteries is happening everywhere else, too. Then there's cardiomyopathy, where the heart muscle itself becomes weak or stiff, often from long-term toxicity -- like the cumulative effect of fluoride, chemotherapy drugs, or even chronic infections like Lyme disease that the medical system refuses to acknowledge. And don't forget valvular heart disease, where the heart's valves get stiff or leaky, usually from years of mineral deficiencies (like magnesium) or infections that were never properly treated. These conditions aren't rare; they're the inevitable result of a lifetime of trusting a system that prioritizes profits over prevention.

Here's the hard truth: these diseases aren't separate. They're all connected by the same root causes -- toxicity, deficiency, and a body pushed to its limits by a world that doesn't value real health. Hypertension damages your arteries, making them prime targets for atherosclerosis, which can then lead to heart attacks, strokes, or heart failure. Arrhythmias can be both a cause and a result of heart failure. And every single one of these conditions is made worse by the very medications prescribed to 'treat' them. Statins deplete CoQ10, weakening your heart. Blood pressure drugs disrupt your electrolytes, setting the stage for arrhythmias. It's a vicious cycle -- and it's entirely by design. The system isn't broken; it's working exactly as intended, keeping you sick and dependent. But you don't have to play along. By understanding these connections, you can interrupt the cycle. Detoxify. Nourish. Move. Breathe clean air. Drink pure water. These aren't just 'lifestyle changes'; they're acts of rebellion against a system that wants you weak and compliant.

Early detection isn't about rushing to the doctor for more tests and drugs; it's about listening to your body and taking action before the damage becomes irreversible. Your body speaks to you in whispers before it screams. That occasional chest tightness. The fatigue after climbing stairs. The dizziness when you stand up too fast. These aren't 'normal signs of aging' -- their warnings. The best diagnostic tools aren't in a hospital; they're in your kitchen, your garden, and your commitment to living in alignment with nature. Start with the basics: eliminate processed foods, which are laced with toxins that inflame your arteries. Test your water for heavy metals and filter it if needed. Sweat regularly -- through exercise or saunas -- to purge the chemicals stored in your fat cells. And perhaps most importantly, question everything. The idea that heart disease is a 'chronic, progressive' condition is a lie. Your heart, like the rest of your body, is designed to heal when given the right conditions. The power to prevent -- and even reverse --cardiovascular disease isn't in a pill. It's in your hands, your choices, and your refusal to accept the status quo.

How Modern Lifestyles Contribute to Heart Disease Epidemics

In the journey to understand cardiovascular disease, it's crucial to examine how our modern lifestyles have become a breeding ground for heart disease epidemics. The shift from traditional to modern lifestyles has been marked by significant changes in diet, physical activity, and stress levels, all of which have profound implications for our heart health. Let's delve into these changes and their impacts, keeping in mind the importance of natural health, personal liberty, and self-reliance.

The modern diet, laden with processed foods, high sugar intake, and unhealthy fats, is a far cry from the wholesome, natural diets of our ancestors. These dietary changes have been linked to obesity and metabolic syndrome, both of which are significant risk factors for cardiovascular disease. Processed foods are often stripped of their natural nutrients and filled with artificial additives, making them a poor choice for maintaining heart health. High sugar intake can lead to insulin resistance, a condition that forces your body to produce more insulin, putting extra stress on your heart. Unhealthy fats, particularly trans fats and excessive saturated fats, can raise your cholesterol levels, increasing your risk of heart disease.

The sedentary behavior that characterizes modern life is another major contributor to heart disease. Prolonged sitting and lack of exercise weaken our cardiovascular system, making it less efficient at pumping blood and delivering oxygen to our bodies. Regular physical activity is essential for maintaining a healthy heart, as it helps control weight, reduces the risk of developing other conditions that may put a strain on the heart, and can help lower blood pressure and cholesterol levels.

Chronic stress and poor sleep patterns are also taking a toll on our cardiovascular health. Chronic stress can lead to hormonal imbalances, such as elevated cortisol levels, which can increase blood pressure and blood sugar levels, both of which are harmful to your heart. Poor sleep patterns, often a result of our fast-paced, always-on lifestyles, can disrupt your body's internal clock, leading to a host of health problems, including heart disease. Quality sleep is crucial for your body to repair and regenerate, and a lack of it can put extra strain on your heart.

Environmental factors, often overlooked, play a significant role in heart health. Air pollution, exposure to electromagnetic fields (EMFs), and chemical toxins can all contribute to heart disease. Air pollution can cause inflammation and damage to your blood vessels, while EMFs can disrupt your body's natural electrical signals, leading to irregular heart rhythms. Chemical toxins, found in everything from our food to our personal care products, can accumulate in our bodies and cause damage to our cardiovascular system.

Social determinants of health, such as socioeconomic status, access to healthcare, and education, also have a significant impact on heart disease. Those with lower socioeconomic status often have less access to healthy foods, safe places to exercise, and quality healthcare, all of which can increase their risk of heart disease. Education, too, plays a crucial role, as it empowers individuals to make informed decisions about their health and navigate the often complex healthcare system.

The rise of heart disease in developing countries adopting Western lifestyles is a stark reminder of the dangers of modern living. As these countries transition from traditional to modern lifestyles, they are seeing a corresponding increase in heart disease rates. This trend underscores the importance of preserving natural, traditional ways of living and the dangers of blindly adopting Western habits.

A comparative analysis of heart disease rates in populations with traditional versus modern lifestyles further highlights the impact of lifestyle on heart health. Populations with traditional lifestyles, characterized by natural diets, regular physical activity, and strong community ties, tend to have lower rates of heart disease. In contrast, populations with modern lifestyles, marked by processed foods, sedentary behavior, and chronic stress, have higher rates of heart disease.

Modern medical practices often focus on symptom management rather than addressing the root causes of heart disease. This approach, while profitable for the pharmaceutical industry, does little to empower individuals to take control of their health. Instead, it fosters a cycle of dependency on medications and healthcare providers, rather than promoting self-reliance and natural health solutions.

In conclusion, the modern lifestyle, with its processed foods, sedentary behavior, chronic stress, and environmental toxins, is a significant contributor to the heart disease epidemic. By understanding these factors and making conscious choices to live more naturally and healthily, we can take control of our heart health and reduce our risk of heart disease. Remember, your health is in your hands, and every choice you make can either contribute to or detract from your well-being.

The Role of Chronic Inflammation in Cardiovascular Decline

Imagine your body as a well-oiled machine, humming along smoothly. Now, picture a silent intruder, a slow-burning fire that doesn't roar but smolders, causing damage over time. This is chronic inflammation, a stealthy saboteur that can wreak havoc on your cardiovascular system, unlike its more noticeable cousin, acute inflammation. Acute inflammation is like a loud alarm, calling attention to an immediate threat, such as a cut or an infection. It's your body's way of saying, 'Hey, I need help here!' But chronic inflammation is different. It's a quiet, persistent hum in the background, a low-grade inflammation that can last for months or even years, often without you even knowing it's there.

Chronic inflammation is like a slow-burning fire that can damage your blood vessels over time. It starts when your body's immune system responds to perceived threats, like poor diet, stress, or environmental toxins. This response can cause your blood vessels to become inflamed, making it easier for plaque to build up and form blockages. This process, known as atherosclerosis, is a major contributor to heart disease. Think of it like a river that slowly gets clogged with debris, making it harder for water to flow. In your body, this 'debris' is made up of fatty substances, cholesterol, cellular waste products, calcium, and other substances that can build up in the inner lining of an artery. Over time, this buildup can narrow the arteries, reducing blood flow and increasing the risk of heart attacks and strokes.

To understand how chronic inflammation affects your heart, let's look at some key players in this process: inflammatory markers. These are like little flags that your body waves to signal that inflammation is present. Three important ones are C-reactive protein (CRP), interleukin-6 (IL-6), and tumor necrosis factor-alpha (TNF-α). High levels of these markers have been linked to an increased risk of cardiovascular disease. CRP, for instance, is produced by the liver in response to inflammation. High levels of HS-CRP can indicate a higher risk of heart disease, even in seemingly healthy individuals. IL-6 and TNF-α are cytokines, which are signaling molecules that mediate and regulate immunity, inflammation, and hematopoiesis. They play crucial roles in both acute and chronic inflammation, and elevated levels of these cytokines have been associated with various chronic diseases, including cardiovascular disease.

So, where does this chronic inflammation come from? It can be triggered by a variety of factors, many of which are within our control. Poor diet, particularly one high in processed foods, sugar, and unhealthy fats, can contribute to chronic inflammation. Stress, both physical and emotional, is another major culprit.

Environmental toxins, such as air pollution and chemicals in our food and water, can also trigger chronic inflammation. Even an imbalance in our gut bacteria, known as gut dysbiosis, can lead to chronic inflammation. It's like having a leaky faucet in your home. If left unchecked, it can cause water damage, mold growth, and structural issues over time. In your body, chronic inflammation can lead to a host of health problems, including cardiovascular disease.

Chronic inflammation doesn't work alone. It often teams up with other risk factors to increase the likelihood of cardiovascular disease. Obesity, for instance, is a major risk factor for heart disease, and it's also associated with chronic inflammation. The same goes for diabetes and hypertension. It's like having multiple bullies ganging up on you. Each one is bad enough on its own, but together, they can cause even more harm. In your body, chronic inflammation can exacerbate the effects of these other risk factors, making it even more important to address inflammation as part of a comprehensive approach to heart health.

One of the key players in the body's inflammatory response is the NLRP3 inflammasome. This is a multi-protein complex that plays a crucial role in the innate immune system. When activated, it triggers the release of inflammatory cytokines, like IL-1β and IL-18, which can contribute to chronic inflammation and cardiovascular disease. Think of the NLRP3 inflammasome like a security system in your body. When it senses danger, it sets off an alarm, calling in reinforcements to deal with the threat. But if this alarm is constantly going off, even when there's no real danger, it can lead to chronic inflammation and damage to your blood vessels.

Understanding the role of the NLRP3 inflammasome in heart disease is crucial, and it's something we'll delve deeper into in Chapter 5.

The good news is that reducing inflammation can help reverse early-stage cardiovascular damage. This can be achieved through a variety of natural approaches, such as improving your diet, managing stress, and reducing your exposure to environmental toxins. For instance, a diet rich in fruits, vegetables, whole grains, and lean proteins can help reduce inflammation. Regular exercise, adequate sleep, and stress management techniques like meditation and yoga can also help keep inflammation in check. It's like giving your body a tune-up, addressing the root causes of inflammation and helping your cardiovascular system run more smoothly.

While conventional anti-inflammatory drugs can help manage inflammation, they often come with a host of side effects and don't address the root causes of inflammation. Natural alternatives, on the other hand, can help reduce inflammation while also promoting overall health. For instance, turmeric, a spice commonly used in Indian cuisine, has potent anti-inflammatory properties. Other natural anti-inflammatories include ginger, green tea, and omega-3 fatty acids found in fish oil. It's like choosing between a quick fix that might cause more problems down the line and a holistic approach that addresses the root causes of inflammation and promotes overall health.

Let me share a story with you about a patient named John. John was a 45-year-old man who came to see me with high blood pressure, high cholesterol, and a family history of heart disease. He was also overweight and had a stressful job. We ran some tests and found that his levels of inflammatory markers, like HS-CRP, were elevated. John was skeptical at first, but he agreed to make some lifestyle changes. He started eating a healthier diet, exercising regularly, and practicing stress management techniques. He also started taking some natural anti-inflammatory supplements, like turmeric and fish oil. Within a few months, John's inflammatory markers had decreased, and his blood pressure and cholesterol levels had improved. He also lost some weight and felt more energetic. John's story is a great example of how addressing chronic inflammation can have a profound impact on heart health.

In conclusion, chronic inflammation is a silent but significant contributor to cardiovascular disease. It's like a slow-burning fire that can damage your blood vessels over time, leading to atherosclerosis and increasing your risk of heart attacks and strokes. But the good news is that there are many natural ways to reduce inflammation and promote heart health. By understanding the role of chronic inflammation in cardiovascular disease, you can take steps to address it and improve your overall health. Remember, your body is like a well-oiled machine. Take care of it, and it will take care of you.

Debunking Myths About Cholesterol and Heart Health

For decades, we've been told that cholesterol is public enemy number one -- a silent killer lurking in our bloodstreams, just waiting to clog our arteries and stop our hearts. The fear campaign has been relentless: eat eggs and you'll drop dead; skip your statin and you're playing Russian roulette with your life. But here's the truth this multi-billion-dollar myth doesn't want you to know: cholesterol isn't the villain it's been made out to be. In fact, it's one of the most vital substances in your body, and the real story about heart health has been buried under layers of corporate greed, bad science, and a medical system that profits more from sickness than from wellness.

Let's start by clearing up the biggest lie of all -- that all cholesterol is harmful. Your body makes cholesterol for a reason, and it's not to kill you. Cholesterol is the raw material for your hormones, including stress-fighting cortisol and sex hormones like testosterone and estrogen. It's a critical component of your brain, making up about 25% of its total cholesterol content, which is why low cholesterol levels are linked to memory problems, depression, and even violent behavior. Cholesterol also keeps your cell membranes flexible and strong, acting like a biological duct tape that holds your cells together. Without it, you wouldn't survive. The idea that cholesterol is some kind of toxic sludge is not just wrong -- it's dangerous. The real question isn't how to eliminate cholesterol, but how to make sure you have the right kinds in the right balance.

Now, let's talk about the so-called 'good' and 'bad' cholesterol -- HDL and LDL. These aren't actually types of cholesterol at all; they're lipoproteins, tiny vehicles that transport cholesterol and fats through your bloodstream. HDL (high-density lipoprotein) is often called 'good' because it helps clear excess cholesterol from your arteries. LDL (low-density lipoprotein), labeled 'bad,' carries cholesterol to your cells where it's needed. But here's what the statin-pushing ads won't tell you: LDL isn't inherently dangerous. The problem arises when LDL particles become small, dense, and oxidized -- damaged by sugar, processed foods, and chronic inflammation. These oxidized LDL particles can embed themselves in your artery walls, triggering plaque formation. Native, unoxidized LDL, on the other hand, is harmless. In fact, some of the healthiest populations on Earth, like the Masai in Africa and the Inuit, have high LDL levels but virtually no heart disease. The issue isn't LDL itself; it's what's happening to it in a toxic, inflammatory environment.

Then there's the myth that eating cholesterol-rich foods like eggs and butter will send your blood cholesterol levels through the roof. This is one of the most persistent lies in nutrition, and it's been thoroughly debunked. Your liver produces about 80% of your body's cholesterol, and when you eat more cholesterol from food, your liver simply makes less. For most people, dietary cholesterol has a minimal impact on blood cholesterol levels. Studies have shown that even when people eat several eggs a day, their cholesterol levels don't skyrocket -- their bodies adjust. The real culprits behind unhealthy cholesterol profiles are refined sugars, processed vegetable oils, and a sedentary lifestyle, not the cholesterol in your omelet. Yet the food industry and pharmaceutical companies have spent decades demonizing eggs and meat while pushing 'heart-healthy' cereals and margarine loaded with sugar and industrial seed oils -- the very things that actually fuel heart disease.

Now, let's tackle the statin scam. Statins are one of the most prescribed drugs in the world, raking in billions for Big Pharma every year. We're told they're a miracle cure, but the reality is far darker. For people who've already had a heart attack, statins might offer some benefit -- but the evidence is weak even there. For everyone else, statins are a disaster. They come with a laundry list of side effects, from muscle pain and weakness to diabetes, cognitive decline, and even increased risk of cancer. Worse, they deplete your body of Coenzyme Q10, a critical nutrient for heart and muscle function, which is why so many people on statins end up with debilitating fatigue and muscle damage. And here's the kicker: statins don't address the root causes of heart disease -- inflammation, oxidative stress, and metabolic dysfunction. They just lower a number on a lab test while your arteries continue to deteriorate. The fact that doctors push these drugs on healthy people as 'preventive medicine' is a testament to how deeply the pharmaceutical industry has infiltrated our healthcare system.

So if cholesterol isn't the real villain, what is? The answer lies in the inflammation hypothesis of heart disease, which has been gaining traction among honest researchers while being ignored by mainstream medicine. Chronic inflammation --driven by poor diet, stress, environmental toxins, and lack of movement --damages your artery walls, making them sticky and prone to plaque buildup.

Oxidized LDL particles get trapped in these damaged areas, and your immune system responds by sending white blood cells to clean up the mess. Over time, this process creates the plaques that can lead to heart attacks. But here's the key: it's not the cholesterol that starts this cascade; it's the inflammation. Countries with high cholesterol levels but low inflammation, like France and Switzerland, have some of the lowest rates of heart disease in the world. Meanwhile, Americans, with our processed food diets and sky-high stress levels, suffer from rampant heart disease despite our obsession with lowering cholesterol.

The cholesterol myth didn't become entrenched by accident. It was a carefully orchestrated campaign driven by conflicts of interest that would make even the most cynical person's head spin. In the 1950s, a researcher named Ancel Keys cherry-picked data from seven countries to 'prove' that dietary fat and cholesterol caused heart disease, while ignoring data from 15 other countries that contradicted his hypothesis. His flawed research became the foundation of the lipid hypothesis, which claimed that saturated fat and cholesterol clog arteries.

Meanwhile, the sugar industry paid scientists to shift the blame away from sugar and onto fat, ensuring that their profits kept rolling in. Pharmaceutical companies jumped on the bandwagon, funding studies that exaggerated the dangers of cholesterol and the benefits of statins. Regulatory agencies like the FDA, heavily influenced by Big Pharma, rubber-stamped these drugs and demonized natural alternatives. The result? A healthcare system that treats cholesterol like a disease instead of a vital substance, while the real causes of heart disease -- sugar, processed foods, and chronic stress -- go unaddressed.

So how do you protect your heart in a world that's been lying to you? First, stop obsessing over your total cholesterol number. What matters far more is the ratio of triglycerides to HDL (aim for below 2:1), the size and density of your LDL particles (large, fluffy LDL is harmless); small, dense LDL is problematic, and markers of inflammation like C-reactive protein (HS-CRPor cardiac CRP). Eat a diet rich in whole, unprocessed foods -- healthy fats from avocados, olive oil, and grass-fed butter; wild-caught fish; organic vegetables; and pastured eggs. Avoid sugar, refined carbs, and processed vegetable oils like the plague. Move your body regularly, manage stress through meditation or time in nature, and prioritize sleep. These lifestyle changes address the root causes of heart disease -- inflammation, oxidative stress, and metabolic dysfunction -- rather than just slapping a Band-Aid on a lab result.

The cholesterol myth is a perfect example of how a corrupt medical system, driven by pharmaceutical profits and government collusion, can hijack our understanding of health. But you don't have to be a victim of this deception. Your body is designed to thrive when given the right tools, and cholesterol is one of those tools -- not a toxin to be feared. By focusing on real food, natural movement, and reducing inflammation, you can achieve heart health that no statin could ever provide. The power to heal lies not in a pill, but in reclaiming the wisdom of how your body truly works. And that's a truth worth fighting for.

The Impact of Stress and Emotional Health on Heart Function

We've all heard the saying, 'Don't let it get to your heart' -- but what if the real danger isn't just metaphorical? Stress doesn't just weigh on your mind; it physically reshapes your heart, your blood vessels, and even the rhythm of your heartbeat. For decades, conventional medicine has treated the heart as a mechanical pump, fixating on cholesterol numbers and blood pressure readings while ignoring the silent, relentless toll of emotional turmoil. Yet the evidence is undeniable: your emotional state is just as critical to heart health as what you eat or how much you exercise. In fact, chronic stress might be the single most overlooked accelerator of cardiovascular disease -- and the key to reversing it lies not in a prescription pad, but in reclaiming control over your mind, your environment, and your emotional resilience.

Let's start with the body's alarm system. When you're under stress -- whether from a traffic jam, a looming deadline, or a global crisis -- your brain triggers the hypothalamic-pituitary-adrenal (HPA) axis, a cascade that floods your system with cortisol and adrenaline. These hormones aren't inherently bad; they're designed to help you fight or flee a threat. But in modern life, the 'threat' is often chronic --endless bills, toxic workplaces, or the 24/7 news cycle designed to keep you in a state of fear. Over time, this hormonal storm raises your blood pressure, spikes your heart rate, and triggers inflammation in your arteries. Cortisol, in particular, damages the delicate lining of your blood vessels (the endothelium), making them stiff and prone to plaque buildup. Meanwhile, adrenaline forces your heart to work harder, like a car engine redlining for years on end. Is it any wonder that long-term stress is linked to a 40% higher risk of heart attack or stroke? The body wasn't built for this kind of marathon.

Then there's the phenomenon of broken heart syndrome -- a stark reminder that emotional pain isn't just 'in your head.' Officially called Takotsubo cardiomyopathy, this condition mimics a heart attack, complete with chest pain and shortness of breath, but it's triggered by sudden, severe emotional stress, like the death of a loved one or a betrayal. Studies show that during these events, the heart's left ventricle temporarily balloons and weakens, as if 'stunned' by the surge of stress hormones. The good news? Most people recover fully.

The bad news? It proves that your heart literally breaks under emotional strain. And while mainstream medicine acknowledges this condition, it rarely connects the dots to everyday stress -- the kind that doesn't knock you down all at once but erodes your heart slowly, like water carving a canyon.

Chronic stress doesn't just wear out your heart; it rewires your brain in ways that make heart disease more likely. Depression and anxiety, for instance, aren't just 'mental health issues' -- they're independent risk factors for cardiovascular disease. Research reveals that people with depression have higher levels of inflammatory markers like C-reactive protein, which accelerates atherosclerosis (the hardening of arteries). Anxiety, meanwhile, disrupts the autonomic nervous system, throwing off the balance between the 'rest-and-digest' parasympathetic branch and the 'fight-or-flight' sympathetic branch. The result? A heart that's constantly revved up, with no time to recover. Neurotransmitters like serotonin and dopamine, often dismissed as 'mood chemicals,' also play a direct role in heart function. Low serotonin levels, for example, are linked to poorer endothelial function -- meaning your blood vessels can't relax and dilate properly. Yet how many cardiologists ask about your emotional well-being during a checkup? The system is broken by design, treating symptoms while ignoring the root cause.

Here's where the medical establishment's failure becomes glaring: it reduces heart health to a handful of biomarkers -- LDL cholesterol, blood pressure, maybe an EKG -- while ignoring the elephant in the room. Heart rate variability (HRV), a measure of the variation in time between heartbeats, is one of the most powerful predictors of cardiovascular health, yet it's rarely discussed in mainstream practice. High HRV means your heart can adapt fluidly to stress; low HRV signals a system stuck in overdrive, unable to bounce back. Studies show that people with low HRV are at significantly higher risk for heart attacks, strokes, and even sudden cardiac death. The kicker? HRV improves with practices like deep breathing, meditation, and spending time in nature -- none of which require a prescription.

But these solutions don't line the pockets of Big Pharma, so they're sidelined in favor of statins and beta-blockers that mask symptoms while the underlying damage continues.

The connection between trauma and heart disease is another blind spot in conventional medicine. Research on survivors of natural disasters, war, or childhood abuse shows that traumatic stress accelerates cardiovascular decline by decades. One study found that women with a history of severe trauma had a 60% higher risk of heart disease than those without -- even after accounting for traditional risk factors like smoking or obesity. Why? Trauma keeps the body locked in a state of hypervigilance, with cortisol levels that never truly return to baseline. Over time, this erodes the cardiovascular system, much like rust eating away at metal. Yet how many doctors ask about your trauma history during a physical? The system isn't just neglectful; it's complicit in keeping you sick by refusing to address the full picture.

Now for the good news: your heart isn't doomed by stress -- it's resilient, and you have more power to protect it than you've been led to believe. Positive emotions like joy, gratitude, and love don't just feel good; they actively heal your heart.

Laughter, for instance, improves endothelial function by 50% -- as much as a brisk walk. Social connection is another potent medicine. Studies show that people with strong social ties have a 50% lower risk of heart disease than those who are isolated. Why? Oxytocin, the 'bonding hormone,' counteracts the damaging effects of cortisol, while shared laughter and touch lower blood pressure and reduce inflammation. Even pets play a role: owning a dog is associated with a 24% reduction in all-cause mortality. These aren't fringe benefits; they're biological necessities that modern life has stripped away -- and reclaiming them is a radical act of self-care.

So what's the solution? First, recognize that stress isn't just 'part of life' -- it's a choice, and you have the power to minimize its grip on you. Start by auditing your environment: Who or what drains your energy? The evening news? A toxic relationship? Social media designed to trigger outrage? Cut it out. Replace it with activities that restore your nervous system -- gardening, forest walks, or even humming (which stimulates the vagus nerve, improving HRV. Prioritize sleep, because poor sleep amplifies cortisol and inflames your arteries. And if you've been told your heart problems are just 'bad genetics' or 'bad luck,' question that narrative. Your body is a self-healing organism, but it needs the right conditions: clean food, clean water, meaningful connections, and a mind free from the constant barrage of fear-based propaganda.

The final piece of the puzzle is this: Your heart doesn't just pump blood -- it responds to your consciousness. Every thought, every emotion, every belief you hold sends a signal to your cardiovascular system. Fear and helplessness constrict; love and empowerment expand. This isn't woolly spirituality -- it's physiology. The heart generates the strongest electromagnetic field in your body, detectable several feet away. When you cultivate coherence -- aligning your heart's rhythm with your breath and emotions -- you don't just reduce stress; you rewrite the script of your health. The medical industrial complex wants you to believe you're a victim of your biology, dependent on their pills and procedures. But the truth is far more liberating: Your heart is waiting for you to take the wheel.

How Environmental Toxins Accelerate Cardiovascular Damage

We live in a world where the air we breathe, the water we drink, and even the products we use daily are laced with invisible threats to our hearts. The truth is, environmental toxins are silently accelerating cardiovascular damage in ways most people never suspect. While mainstream medicine pushes pills and procedures, the real culprits -- heavy metals, synthetic chemicals, and electromagnetic pollution --

are ignored or downplayed by institutions that profit from sickness. But once you understand how these toxins work, you can take powerful steps to protect your heart and reclaim your health.

The list of common environmental toxins harming cardiovascular health is longer than most realize. Heavy metals like lead, mercury, and cadmium lurk in contaminated water, dental fillings, and even some foods. Lead, for example, has been linked to hypertension and atherosclerosis by disrupting the delicate balance of nitric oxide, a molecule critical for healthy blood flow. Mercury, often found in fish and dental amalgams, promotes oxidative stress -- a process that damages blood vessels and sets the stage for heart disease. Cadmium, a byproduct of industrial pollution and cigarette smoke, accumulates in the kidneys and arteries, stiffening blood vessels and raising blood pressure over time. Pesticides, another pervasive threat, don't just poison pests -- they poison people. Studies show that long-term exposure to herbicides like glyphosate (the active ingredient in Roundup) is associated with higher rates of heart failure and irregular heartbeats. And let's not forget air pollutants, which are far more dangerous than most health authorities admit. The smaller the particle, the deeper it penetrates -- PM2.5, microscopic specks of pollution from vehicle exhaust and industrial emissions, slip past lung defenses, enter the bloodstream, and trigger systemic inflammation that directly harms the heart.

Then there are endocrine-disrupting chemicals like bisphenol A (BPA) and phthalates, found in plastics, food packaging, and personal care products. These synthetic compounds mimic hormones, throwing off the body's natural signaling systems. BPA, for instance, interferes with estrogen receptors, promoting inflammation in the arterial walls and increasing the risk of plaque buildup.

Phthalates, often hidden in fragrances and vinyl products, have been tied to higher blood pressure and insulin resistance -- both key players in cardiovascular decline. The tragedy? These chemicals are everywhere, from water bottles to shampoos, and regulatory agencies have done little to protect the public. Instead, they've allowed corporations to flood the market with toxins while downplaying the risks.

Air pollution deserves special attention because its impact on heart health is both immediate and long-term. Particulate matter (PM2.5) and nitrogen oxides from traffic and factories don't just irritate the lungs -- they set off a cascade of damage in the cardiovascular system. When these pollutants enter the bloodstream, they trigger oxidative stress, a process where free radicals attack cells, including those lining blood vessels. Over time, this leads to endothelial dysfunction, where arteries lose their flexibility and become prone to clogging. Research confirms that long-term exposure to high levels of PM2.5 increases the risk of heart attacks, strokes, and even fatal arrhythmias. Yet, instead of addressing the root cause --industrial pollution and poor urban planning -- governments and health agencies focus on symptom management, pushing statins and blood pressure drugs while ignoring the toxic environment that's making people sick in the first place.

Smoking and secondhand smoke remain among the most preventable yet persistent cardiovascular toxins. Cigarette smoke contains thousands of chemicals, including heavy metals and carcinogens, that directly damage the heart and blood vessels. Nicotine raises blood pressure and heart rate, while carbon monoxide robs tissues of oxygen, forcing the heart to work harder.

Secondhand smoke is just as dangerous, exposing nonsmokers to the same oxidative stress and endothelial damage. The solution? Avoidance. But in a world where smoking is still glamorized and vaping is marketed as "harmless," many remain unaware of the silent toll it takes on their hearts. The truth is, no amount of tobacco exposure is safe -- and the cardiovascular system pays the price long before cancer ever develops.

Electromagnetic fields (EMFs) from wireless devices, power lines, and 5G networks are another underappreciated threat to heart health. While mainstream science often dismisses concerns about EMFs as "conspiracy theories," independent research tells a different story. Prolonged exposure to high-frequency electromagnetic radiation can disrupt the heart's electrical signaling, leading to arrhythmias and elevated blood pressure. Studies have shown that people living near power lines or cell towers have higher rates of hypertension and irregular heartbeats. Even everyday devices like smartphones and Wi-Fi routers emit EMFs that may contribute to chronic stress on the cardiovascular system. The solution isn't to live in a Faraday cage, but to minimize exposure -- turning off Wi-Fi at night, using wired connections when possible, and keeping phones away from the body.

One of the most insidious aspects of environmental toxins is bioaccumulation --the process by which toxins build up in the body over time. Heavy metals, pesticides, and industrial chemicals don't just pass through; they settle into tissues, organs, and bones, where they slowly wreak havoc. Lead, for example, can remain in the body for decades, continuously damaging blood vessels and nerves. Mercury binds to fatty tissues, including those in the brain and heart, disrupting cellular function. The result? A gradual but steady decline in cardiovascular health, often misdiagnosed as "normal aging" or "genetic bad luck." Detoxification --through nutrition, sweating, and binders like activated charcoal or zeolite -- can help reverse this buildup, but prevention is always the best strategy. Eating organic, filtering water, and choosing non-toxic personal care products are simple yet powerful ways to reduce your toxic load.

The good news is that reducing toxin exposure can lead to dramatic improvements in heart health. Take the case of Mark, a 52-year-old man with high blood pressure, fatigue, and occasional chest tightness. After testing revealed elevated levels of lead and cadmium, he made sweeping changes: switching to filtered water, eating organic foods, and replacing his plastic containers with glass. Within six months, his blood pressure normalized, his energy returned, and his follow-up tests showed significantly lower metal levels. His story isn't unique --countless people have reversed cardiovascular symptoms by addressing their toxic burden. The key is awareness and action. Most doctors won't test for heavy metals or endocrine disruptors unless you ask, and even then, they're quick to dismiss the results. But when you take control of your environment, you take control of your heart health.

So what can you do today to protect your heart from environmental toxins? Start with the basics: drink filtered water to avoid heavy metals and chlorine, eat organic to reduce pesticide exposure, and choose natural personal care products free of phthalates and parabens. Open windows to improve indoor air quality, but use an air purifier if you live in a high-pollution area. Limit plastic use, especially for food storage, and opt for glass or stainless steel. Reduce EMF exposure by keeping devices away from your body and turning off Wi-Fi at night. And if you smoke or vape, quit -- your heart will thank you faster than you think. The reality is, we're all exposed to toxins daily, but the degree of exposure -- and the resulting damage -- is within your control. By making conscious choices, you can shield your heart from the silent assault of environmental pollutants and build a foundation for lasting cardiovascular health.

The Connection Between Metabolic Health and Heart Disease

In our journey to understand cardiovascular disease, we must shine a light on a crucial yet often overlooked factor: metabolic health. Metabolic health is not just about maintaining a healthy weight; it's about how well your body processes food into energy, manages blood sugar, and maintains healthy levels of fats in your blood. The key components of metabolic health include blood sugar control, insulin sensitivity, lipid profile, blood pressure, and waist circumference. These factors are not just numbers on a lab report; they are vital signs that indicate how well your body is functioning at a cellular level.

Insulin resistance and metabolic syndrome are like silent saboteurs, quietly driving cardiovascular disease through inflammation, oxidative stress, and endothelial dysfunction. When your body becomes resistant to insulin, it's like having a broken thermostat that can't properly regulate your blood sugar. This leads to a cascade of problems, including chronic inflammation and damage to the lining of your blood vessels, which can ultimately result in heart disease.

Metabolic syndrome, a cluster of conditions that occur together, increases your risk of heart disease, stroke, and type 2 diabetes. It's a perfect storm of high blood pressure, high blood sugar, excess body fat around the waist, and abnormal cholesterol levels.

Visceral fat, the fat stored deep within your abdominal cavity, is not just an innocent bystander. It's an active player in producing inflammatory cytokines and disrupting metabolic function. These inflammatory molecules can wreak havoc on your body, promoting insulin resistance and damaging your blood vessels. The more visceral fat you have, the higher your risk of developing metabolic syndrome and cardiovascular disease. It's like having a factory of inflammation right in the middle of your body, constantly churning out harmful substances.

The link between type 2 diabetes and heart disease is well-established, with a condition known as 'diabetic cardiomyopathy' serving as a stark reminder of this connection. Diabetic cardiomyopathy refers to the ability of diabetes to cause heart disease independently of other risk factors like high blood pressure or coronary artery disease. High blood sugar levels can damage your blood vessels and the nerves that control your heart, leading to a host of cardiovascular problems. It's a sobering thought, but it also underscores the importance of managing your blood sugar levels to protect your heart.

High-fructose corn syrup and refined carbohydrates are like wolves in sheep's clothing, masquerading as food while wreaking havoc on your metabolic health and increasing your risk of heart disease. These substances can lead to rapid spikes in blood sugar, promote insulin resistance, and contribute to the development of visceral fat. They are often hidden in processed foods, making it all too easy to consume them unknowingly. By choosing whole, unprocessed foods, you can take a significant step towards improving your metabolic health and protecting your heart.

The gut microbiome, the community of microorganisms living in your digestive tract, plays a crucial role in metabolic health and cardiovascular function. These tiny organisms help digest food, produce vitamins, and regulate your immune system. An imbalance in your gut microbiome can lead to inflammation, insulin resistance, and other metabolic problems. It's a fascinating and complex ecosystem, and taking care of it through a healthy diet and lifestyle can have profound benefits for your heart and overall health.

Conventional metrics like Body Mass Index (BMI) have limitations and can be misleading. They don't tell the whole story about your metabolic health. Instead, metabolic markers like fasting insulin and HbA1c provide a more accurate picture. Fasting insulin measures how much insulin is in your blood after a period of not eating, while HbA1c reflects your average blood sugar levels over the past two to three months. These markers can give you and your healthcare provider valuable insights into your metabolic health and risk of heart disease.

Improving metabolic health can reverse early-stage heart disease, offering a beacon of hope for those looking to take control of their health. By addressing insulin resistance, reducing visceral fat, and improving blood sugar control, you can make significant strides in protecting and even healing your heart. It's never too late to start making positive changes, and the benefits can be profound and life-changing.

Conventional dietary guidelines that promote high-carbohydrate, low-fat diets have contributed to the metabolic health crisis we face today. These guidelines, often influenced by corporate interests and outdated science, have led many astray, promoting a diet that can exacerbate insulin resistance and metabolic syndrome. By questioning these guidelines and seeking out independent, evidence-based health information, you can make informed decisions about your diet and take a significant step towards improving your metabolic health and protecting your heart.

In our quest to understand and prevent cardiovascular disease, we must not overlook the crucial role of metabolic health. By taking a holistic, informed approach to our health, we can protect ourselves from the silent saboteurs of insulin resistance and metabolic syndrome. Remember, your health is in your hands, and every positive change you make is a step towards a healthier, happier heart.

Why Conventional Medicine Fails in Long-Term Heart Disease Prevention

Let's dive into why conventional medicine often falls short when it comes to preventing heart disease in the long run. The main issue is that it tends to focus on managing symptoms rather than addressing the root causes of the problem. Instead of looking at the big picture and trying to figure out why someone might be developing heart disease, doctors often just prescribe medications to lower blood pressure or cholesterol. This approach might make the numbers look better on paper, but it doesn't necessarily make the patient any healthier overall.

One of the biggest problems is the overreliance on pharmaceuticals like statins, beta-blockers, and blood pressure medications. While these drugs can be helpful in the short term, they often come with a host of side effects and don't do much to actually prevent heart disease from progressing. For example, statins might lower your cholesterol numbers, but they don't address the underlying inflammation and metabolic issues that are often at the heart of cardiovascular problems. Plus, many of these medications can cause nutrient depletions and other issues that can actually make your health worse in the long run.

Another major issue is the conflicts of interest that are rampant in medical research. So much of the research that guides treatment decisions is funded by pharmaceutical companies, which obviously have a vested interest in selling more drugs. This can lead to biased studies and treatment guidelines that push medications over more natural, preventive approaches. It's hard to trust the system when the people making the recommendations stand to profit from those very recommendations.

The way our healthcare system is set up also incentivizes procedures and medications over actual preventive care. In a fee-for-service model, doctors and hospitals make more money by doing more tests and procedures, not by keeping people healthy. This means there's not much motivation to spend time counseling patients on lifestyle changes that could actually prevent heart disease from developing in the first place. It's a sad reality that our healthcare system often profits more from sickness than from wellness.

Perhaps one of the most glaring problems is the lack of emphasis on lifestyle interventions in conventional medical training and practice. Most doctors just don't have the time or the training to really delve into nutrition, stress management, or other lifestyle factors that play a huge role in heart health. They're taught to treat diseases with drugs and procedures, not to prevent them with diet and lifestyle changes. This is a huge disservice to patients who could benefit immensely from these approaches.

When you look at the data, it's clear that conventional approaches aren't doing enough to reduce heart disease mortality rates. Despite all the medications and procedures, heart disease remains the leading cause of death worldwide. This should be a wake-up call that what we're doing isn't working as well as it should be. We need to start looking at alternative approaches and focusing more on prevention rather than just treatment.

Medical dogma also plays a big role in resisting alternative approaches to heart disease prevention. For years, we've been told that cholesterol is the enemy and that lowering it with statins is the key to heart health. But this lipid hypothesis has been increasingly called into question, with many experts now recognizing that cholesterol is just one small piece of a much larger puzzle. Unfortunately, the medical establishment is often slow to change, and many doctors are still stuck in this outdated way of thinking.

Conventional medicine also tends to overlook important factors like environmental toxins, chronic stress, and metabolic health when it comes to heart disease prevention. These are all huge contributors to cardiovascular problems, but they're often ignored in favor of a more narrow focus on things like cholesterol and blood pressure. We can't expect to make real progress in preventing heart disease if we're not addressing all of the factors that contribute to it.

So what's the solution? We need a more integrative and preventive approach to cardiovascular health. This means looking at the whole person, not just their cholesterol numbers. It means addressing lifestyle factors like diet, exercise, stress management, and environmental toxins. And it means being open to alternative approaches that might not be part of conventional medical dogma but have shown promise in preventing and even reversing heart disease. It's time for a change in how we approach heart health, and that change needs to start with a focus on prevention and true healing, not just symptom management.

In the end, it's about empowering individuals to take control of their own health. This means providing them with the information and tools they need to make real, lasting changes in their lives. It's not about just popping a pill and hoping for the best. It's about making informed decisions, addressing root causes, and working towards true wellness. This is the future of heart disease prevention, and it's a future that we should all be striving for.

2: Natural Prevention Strategies for Heart Health

Imagine walking through a lush garden, plucking ripe berries from the vine, cracking open nuts fresh from the tree, and pulling vibrant greens straight from the earth. Now contrast that with tearing open a plastic package filled with ingredients you can't pronounce, manufactured in a factory hundreds of miles away. The difference isn't just about taste -- it's about the very foundation of heart health. Whole foods, the way nature intended them, hold the key to protecting your heart in ways no processed meal or pharmaceutical ever could. And the best part? You don't need a prescription, a doctor's approval, or a corporate middleman to access their power.

Whole foods are exactly what they sound like: foods in their natural, unrefined state, untouched by industrial processing. Think of an apple with its skin still intact, a handful of almonds straight from the shell, or a fillet of wild-caught salmon. These foods are packed with nutrients -- vitamins, minerals, fiber, and phytonutrients -- that work together like a well-rehearsed orchestra. Processed foods, on the other hand, are like that same orchestra after half the musicians have been replaced with robots programmed to play only one note. They're stripped of their natural complexity, pumped full of synthetic additives, and designed to sit on a shelf for months without spoiling. Your heart doesn't want preservatives, artificial flavors, or high-fructose corn syrup -- it wants the real thing. And when you give it real food, it rewards you with strength, resilience, and longevity.

Let's talk about the superstars of the whole foods world when it comes to heart health. Leafy greens like kale, spinach, and Swiss chard are packed with magnesium, a mineral that helps regulate blood pressure and keeps your heart rhythm steady. Berries -- blueberries, strawberries, raspberries -- are bursting with antioxidants that fight inflammation, one of the silent killers of heart disease. Nuts and seeds, from walnuts to flaxseeds, deliver heart-healthy fats that lower bad cholesterol and keep your arteries flexible. Fatty fish like salmon and sardines are rich in omega-3s, which reduce triglycerides and prevent dangerous blood clots.

And don't forget whole grains like quinoa, brown rice, and oats, which provide fiber that sweeps cholesterol out of your body like a broom. These aren't just foods; they're medicine, grown by the earth and delivered straight to your plate.

What makes whole foods so powerful isn't just the individual nutrients they contain -- it's how those nutrients work together. Science calls this synergy, and it's something no lab-made supplement or fortified cereal can replicate. For example, the vitamin C in an orange doesn't just sit there by itself; it's paired with flavonoids and fiber that help your body absorb and use it more effectively. The lycopene in tomatoes is far more bioavailable when you eat the whole tomato than when you take it in pill form. And the combination of healthy fats, fiber, and antioxidants in a handful of almonds does more to protect your heart than any single ingredient could on its own. Nature doesn't do isolation -- it does harmony. When you eat whole foods, you're not just feeding your body; you're giving it a symphony of nutrients designed to work in perfect balance.

Oxidative stress and inflammation are like the rust and corrosion eating away at your heart's machinery. Every day, your body is bombarded with free radicals -- unstable molecules that damage cells and accelerate aging. Processed foods, pollution, and even stress add fuel to this fire. But whole foods are your body's fire extinguishers. The antioxidants in colorful fruits and vegetables -- like the deep purple of blackberries or the bright orange of carrots -- neutralize free radicals before they can do harm. Turmeric, ginger, and garlic pack anti-inflammatory punches that calm the fires of chronic inflammation, which is at the root of nearly every heart-related problem, from atherosclerosis to high blood pressure. When you eat a diet rich in whole foods, you're essentially arming your body with an internal cleanup crew, sweeping away the debris that clogs your arteries and weakens your heart.

If you're looking for a real-world example of how whole foods can transform heart health, look no further than the Mediterranean diet. This isn't some fad created by a food corporation; it's a way of eating that's been perfected over centuries by people who live in regions where heart disease is practically unheard of. The Mediterranean diet is built on whole foods: olive oil instead of butter, fresh fish instead of processed meats, and plenty of vegetables, fruits, nuts, and legumes.

Study after study has shown that people who follow this diet have lower rates of heart attacks, strokes, and high cholesterol. They also live longer, healthier lives --without relying on a pharmacy's worth of pills. The beauty of it? There's no patent on olive oil or fresh herbs. No corporation controls the rights to eat a handful of walnuts or a bowl of lentils. This is health that's accessible to everyone, no middleman required.

Now, let's address the elephant in the room: cost. It's true that a bag of organic apples might cost more than a box of frozen pizza. But here's the thing -- what's the real cost of that pizza? When you factor in the long-term expenses of doctor visits, medications, and lost quality of life, those "cheap" processed foods start to look pretty expensive. The good news is, eating whole foods doesn't have to break the bank. Buy in bulk, choose seasonal produce, and grow what you can -- even a small herb garden on your windowsill can make a difference. Farmers' markets often have better prices than grocery stores, especially toward the end of the day when vendors are looking to sell their last batches. And remember, every whole food meal you eat is an investment in a future without hospital bills or pharmaceutical dependencies.

One of the biggest barriers people face when switching to whole foods is convenience. In a world where drive-thrus and microwave dinners are the norm, taking the time to chop vegetables or soak beans can feel like a luxury. But here's a secret: whole foods can be just as convenient -- you just need a little strategy.

Spend a couple of hours on the weekend prepping meals for the week. Cook big batches of grains and roast trays of vegetables so you can mix and match them throughout the week. Keep healthy snacks like nuts, dried fruit, and cut-up veggies within easy reach. And if you're short on time, focus on simple meals that don't require a recipe: a bowl of oatmeal topped with berries and seeds, a salad with whatever greens and proteins you have on hand, or a smoothie blended with frozen fruit and spinach. The more you do it, the easier it gets -- and the better you'll feel.

Let me tell you about Carlos, a 58-year-old man who came to me after his doctor told him he was on the fast track to a heart attack. His cholesterol was through the roof, his blood pressure was dangerously high, and he was taking three different medications just to keep things under control. Carlos had grown up eating the standard American diet -- lots of meat, dairy, and processed foods -- and he didn't see how he could possibly change. But after his grandson was born, he decided he wanted to be around to watch the kid grow up. So we started small: swapping his morning cereal for oatmeal with flaxseeds and blueberries, replacing his lunch deli sandwich with a big salad loaded with veggies and chickpeas, and trading his evening chips for a handful of almonds and an apple. Within three months, his cholesterol dropped by 40 points, his blood pressure normalized, and his doctor took him off one of his medications. A year later, Carlos was medication-free, had lost 25 pounds, and was growing his own herbs and tomatoes in his backyard. His story isn't unique -- it's what happens when you give your body the tools it needs to heal itself.

The final piece of the puzzle is sourcing your food wisely. Organic and locally grown foods aren't just better for the environment -- they're better for you. Conventionally grown produce is often sprayed with pesticides that disrupt your hormones, damage your gut, and contribute to inflammation. Animals raised in factory farms are pumped full of antibiotics and growth hormones that end up in your body when you eat them. By choosing organic, you're reducing your toxic load and giving your heart one less thing to fight against. And when you buy local, you're not just supporting your community -- you're getting food that's fresher, more nutrient-dense, and hasn't been sitting in a truck for weeks losing its vitality. If organic isn't an option, focus on the "Clean 15" -- the fruits and vegetables that tend to have the lowest pesticide residues. Every small choice adds up to a bigger impact on your health.

At the end of the day, the power of whole foods isn't just about preventing heart disease -- it's about reclaiming your health from a system that wants to keep you sick and dependent. Big Pharma doesn't profit when you eat a salad instead of taking a statin. The processed food industry doesn't thrive when you cook from scratch instead of buying their pre-packaged meals. But you thrive. Your heart thrives. And that's what matters. So next time you're standing in the grocery store aisle, faced with the choice between a box of crackers and a bunch of carrots, remember: every bite is a vote. A vote for your health, your freedom, and your future. Choose wisely -- your heart is counting on you.

REFERENCES:

- *Gonzalez, Michael J., Jorge R. Miranda Massari, and Andrew W. Saul. I Have Cancer.*
- *Mozaffarian, Dariush. Eat Fat, Get Thin: Why the Fat We Eat Is the Key to Sustained Weight Loss and Vibrant Health.*
- *Hyman, Mark. The Blood Sugar Solution: The UltraHealthy Program for Losing Weight, Preventing Disease, and Feeling Great Now!*
- *Campbell, T. Colin, and Thomas M. Campbell. The China Study: The Most Comprehensive Study of Nutrition Ever Conducted and the Startling Implications for Diet, Weight Loss, and Long-Term Health.*
- *Esselstyn, Caldwell B. Prevent and Reverse Heart Disease: The Revolutionary, Scientifically Proven, Nutrition-Based Cure.*

Essential Nutrients and Supplements for a Strong Heart

In a world where mainstream medicine often overlooks the power of natural solutions, it's empowering to know that we can take control of our heart health with essential nutrients and supplements. Let's dive into the key players that can make a real difference in keeping your heart strong and resilient.

Magnesium is a mineral that often doesn't get the attention it deserves. It's crucial for maintaining healthy blood pressure levels and supporting overall cardiovascular function. When we're deficient in magnesium, our blood vessels can become constricted, making it harder for our hearts to do their job efficiently. Food sources like leafy greens, nuts, and seeds are excellent, but many of us may benefit from supplementation to reach optimal levels.

Potassium is another essential mineral that works hand in hand with magnesium. It helps regulate your heartbeat and supports healthy blood pressure. When potassium levels are low, it can lead to heart palpitations and other cardiovascular issues. Bananas are often touted as a great source, but did you know that sweet potatoes and spinach actually contain more potassium per serving? It's always best to get your nutrients from a variety of whole food sources.

CoQ10, or coenzyme Q10, is a powerful antioxidant that plays a vital role in mitochondrial energy production. Our mitochondria are like tiny power plants within our cells, and CoQ10 helps them generate the energy our hearts need to function optimally. As we age, our natural CoQ10 levels decline, which is why supplementation can be particularly beneficial for those over 40. It's also been shown to support healthy blood pressure and overall cardiovascular function.

Omega-3 fatty acids, found in fatty fish like salmon and mackerel, as well as in flaxseeds and walnuts, are essential for heart health. They help reduce triglycerides, support healthy blood pressure, and may even help prevent arterial plaque buildup. If you're not a fan of fish, high-quality fish oil or algae-based supplements can be a great alternative. Just be sure to choose a supplement that's been third-party tested for purity and potency.

Vitamin K2 is a lesser-known but incredibly important nutrient for heart health. It works synergistically with vitamins D and A to help prevent arterial calcification, a condition where calcium builds up in the arteries, making them stiff and inflexible. This is crucial because many people take calcium supplements without realizing that without adequate vitamin K2, that calcium may not be properly utilized and could end up in the wrong places, like our arteries. Fermented foods like natto are rich in K2, but supplementation may be necessary for optimal levels.

It's essential to understand that nutrients don't work in isolation. They rely on each other for proper absorption and function. For example, magnesium helps activate vitamin D, and vitamin D enhances calcium absorption. This nutrient synergy is why it's so important to focus on a balanced, whole-foods-based approach to heart health. When we're deficient in one nutrient, it can create a domino effect, impacting the function of others.

While synthetic supplements can provide some benefits, they often pale in comparison to whole-food-based supplements. Our bodies are designed to recognize and utilize nutrients in their natural forms, complete with the cofactors and enzymes that support their absorption and function. When we isolate nutrients in synthetic forms, they may not be as effectively utilized by our bodies.

This is why I always recommend choosing whole-food-based supplements whenever possible.

Adaptogenic herbs like ashwagandha and rhodiola can also play a supportive role in heart health, particularly when it comes to managing stress. Chronic stress takes a toll on our cardiovascular system, and these herbs can help our bodies adapt and respond more resiliently. They've been used for centuries in traditional medicine systems and are gaining recognition in the modern world for their heart-protective benefits.

When choosing supplements, quality is key. Look for products that have been third-party tested for purity and potency. This means that an independent lab has verified that what's on the label is actually in the bottle and that it's free from contaminants. Additionally, consider the sourcing of the ingredients. Are they from high-quality, organic sources? Are they sustainably harvested? These factors can make a big difference in the effectiveness of the supplement.

It's important to address some common misconceptions about supplements. First and foremost, supplements are not a replacement for a healthy diet. They are meant to complement and support your nutritional intake, not take the place of whole, nutrient-dense foods. Additionally, more is not always better when it comes to supplementation. It's essential to work with a healthcare practitioner knowledgeable in natural medicine to determine the right doses and combinations for your unique needs.

To give you a practical starting point, here's a sample supplement protocol for supporting heart health. For general maintenance, consider a high-quality multivitamin that includes activated B vitamins, magnesium, and a blend of antioxidants. Add in a separate omega-3 supplement, aiming for a combined EPA and DHA dose of around 1,000 mg per day. If you're over 40 or have specific heart health concerns, you may benefit from adding CoQ10 (100-200 mg per day) and vitamin K2 (100-200 mcg per day). Always remember to consult with a healthcare practitioner before starting any new supplement regimen, especially if you have existing health conditions or are taking medications.

In our journey towards optimal heart health, it's empowering to know that we have natural tools at our disposal. By focusing on essential nutrients and high-quality supplements, we can support our cardiovascular system in a way that aligns with our bodies' innate wisdom. As with any health endeavor, listen to your body, work with trusted healthcare practitioners, and always prioritize a balanced, whole-foods-based approach. Your heart will thank you for it.

In the next section, we'll explore the profound impact that stress has on our heart health and delve into natural strategies for managing stress and supporting emotional well-being. After all, a strong heart is not just about the physical aspects; our emotional and mental states play a significant role as well. So, let's continue our journey towards a healthier, happier heart.

How Intermittent Fasting and Time-Restricted Eating Protect the Heart

Imagine your heart as a well-tuned engine, humming along smoothly when given the right fuel at the right times. Now picture what happens when that engine is constantly flooded with fuel -- it sputters, clogs, and eventually wears down. That's what happens to our hearts when we eat around the clock, never giving our bodies a chance to rest, repair, and reset. Intermittent fasting (IF) and time-restricted eating (TRE) are like hitting the reset button for your heart, offering it the break it desperately needs in a world that tells us to eat all day, every day.

These aren't just diet trends; they're ancient, time-tested practices that align with how our bodies were designed to function -- long before processed foods, 24/7 snacking, and pharmaceutical quick fixes took over.

Intermittent fasting and time-restricted eating are often used interchangeably, but they're not quite the same. Intermittent fasting is the broader term, referring to any eating pattern that cycles between periods of eating and fasting. This could mean fasting for a full 24 hours once or twice a week, or it might involve more structured approaches like the 5:2 method, where you eat normally for five days and drastically reduce calories for two non-consecutive days. Time-restricted eating, on the other hand, is a type of intermittent fasting where you confine all your eating to a specific window each day -- most commonly 8 hours -- followed by a 16-hour fast. For example, you might eat between noon and 8 p.m., then fast until noon the next day. Both methods work with your body's natural rhythms instead of against them, giving your digestive system a much-needed break and allowing your body to tap into its own healing mechanisms.

One of the most powerful ways fasting protects your heart is by improving insulin sensitivity. When you eat constantly, your body is in a perpetual state of processing glucose, which can lead to insulin resistance -- a major driver of heart disease. Fasting, however, gives your body a chance to burn through stored glucose and start using fat for energy instead. This shift not only helps stabilize blood sugar levels but also reduces inflammation, which is at the root of nearly every chronic disease, including cardiovascular disease. Studies have shown that intermittent fasting can lower markers of inflammation like hs-

C-reactive protein (hs-CRP), which is strongly linked to heart attacks and strokes. It's like giving your body a chance to cool down an engine that's been running too hot for too long.

Fasting also promotes something called autophagy, a process where your cells essentially clean house, breaking down and recycling damaged components.

Think of it as your body's internal recycling program. When autophagy is working well, it helps clear out the cellular junk that can contribute to plaque buildup in your arteries and other heart-related issues. This process is particularly important for mitochondrial health -- the mitochondria are the powerhouses of your cells, and when they're functioning optimally, your heart has the energy it needs to keep beating strongly. Poor mitochondrial function, on the other hand, is linked to heart failure and other cardiovascular problems. By enhancing autophagy, fasting helps keep your mitochondria -- and by extension, your heart -- in top shape.

Another key benefit of fasting is its ability to reduce visceral fat, the dangerous fat that wraps around your organs, including your heart. Unlike the fat you can pinch under your skin, visceral fat is metabolically active, pumping out inflammatory chemicals that damage your arteries and increase your risk of heart disease.

Fasting helps your body shift from burning glucose to burning fat, and over time, this can significantly reduce visceral fat stores. Research has shown that time-restricted eating, in particular, can lead to a reduction in waist circumference -- a good indicator that visceral fat is being lost -- without the need for calorie counting or extreme dieting. It's a natural, sustainable way to protect your heart by targeting one of its biggest enemies.

Fasting doesn't just help you lose fat; it also improves your lipid profile, which is a fancy way of saying it helps balance your cholesterol and triglyceride levels. High triglycerides and low HDL (the "good" cholesterol) are both risk factors for heart disease, and fasting has been shown to improve both. For example, studies on time-restricted eating have found that participants experience reductions in LDL (the "bad" cholesterol) and triglycerides, along with increases in HDL. This is huge because cholesterol-lowering drugs, which are pushed by the pharmaceutical industry, come with a host of side effects and don't address the root causes of poor lipid profiles. Fasting, on the other hand, tackles the problem at its source by improving how your body processes and stores fats.

Blood pressure is another area where fasting shines. High blood pressure, or hypertension, is often called the silent killer because it damages your arteries over time without you even realizing it. Fasting helps lower blood pressure by improving endothelial function -- the health of the cells that line your blood vessels. When your endothelial cells are healthy, they produce nitric oxide, a molecule that helps your blood vessels relax and dilate, reducing blood pressure. Poor endothelial function, on the other hand, is a hallmark of heart disease.

Fasting also reduces oxidative stress, which is another factor that can damage your blood vessels and lead to hypertension. By supporting endothelial health and reducing oxidative stress, fasting helps keep your blood pressure in a healthy range naturally, without the need for medications that often come with harmful side effects.

If you're new to fasting, the idea of going without food for extended periods might seem daunting, but it's easier than you think -- especially when you start small. A simple way to begin is with a 12-hour fast overnight. For example, if you finish dinner by 7 p.m., you'd wait until 7 a.m. the next morning to eat breakfast. Once you're comfortable with that, you can gradually increase your fasting window to 14 or 16 hours, which is where many people see the most benefits. The 16:8 method -- fasting for 16 hours and eating within an 8-hour window -- is one of the most popular and sustainable approaches. Another option is the 5:2 method, where you eat normally for five days and then consume about 500-600 calories on two nonconsecutive days. The key is to find a rhythm that works for your lifestyle and stick with it. Remember, your body is designed to handle periods without food; it's only in our modern world of constant snacking that we've forgotten this natural ability.

Of course, fasting isn't for everyone, and it's important to listen to your body. If you have a history of disordered eating, fasting might not be a good fit, as it could trigger unhealthy patterns. Similarly, if you're pregnant, breastfeeding, or dealing with certain medical conditions like diabetes (especially if you're on medication, you should approach fasting with caution and ideally under the guidance of a healthcare provider who understands natural health. Some people also worry about losing muscle or feeling low on energy when they fast, but these concerns are often overblown. As long as you're eating enough protein during your eating windows and staying hydrated, your body will hold onto muscle. And while you might feel a bit sluggish at first as your body adapts to burning fat for fuel, most people actually report having more steady energy once they're fat-adapted.

Let's look at a real-life example to see how powerful fasting can be. Take the case of Mark, a 52-year-old man who came to me with high blood pressure, elevated triglycerides, and a family history of heart disease. He was on the verge of being put on statins and blood pressure medication, but he wanted to try a natural approach first. We started him on a 16:8 time-restricted eating plan, where he ate between 11 a.m. and 7 p.m. each day. Within three months, his triglycerides dropped by 40%, his HDL increased, and his blood pressure normalized. He also lost 15 pounds, most of it around his midsection, which is a clear sign he was shedding visceral fat. What's more, he reported feeling more energetic and mentally clear than he had in years. Mark's story isn't unique; it's a testament to how our bodies are designed to heal when given the right conditions. Fasting isn't about deprivation -- it's about giving your body the space it needs to thrive.

In a world where the pharmaceutical industry profits from keeping people sick and dependent on medications, fasting offers a refreshing alternative -- a way to take control of your health using the tools your body already has. It's free, it's natural, and it works with your biology instead of against it. Whether you're looking to prevent heart disease or reverse early signs of trouble, intermittent fasting and time-restricted eating are powerful strategies that put you back in the driver's seat. And the best part? You don't need a prescription, a doctor's approval, or a expensive supplement to get started. All you need is the willingness to press pause on the constant eating and let your body do what it was designed to do: heal itself.

The Role of Physical Activity in Maintaining Cardiovascular Resilience

There's a quiet revolution happening in heart health, and it doesn't come in a prescription bottle. For decades, we've been told that managing cardiovascular disease means relying on pharmaceuticals, invasive procedures, and a system that profits from keeping people sick. But the truth is far simpler -- and far more empowering. The human body is designed to thrive when given the right conditions, and one of the most powerful tools we have to protect our hearts is something we've had all along: movement. Not the kind forced on us by gym memberships or fitness trends, but the kind that aligns with how our ancestors lived -- active, engaged, and free from the sedentary traps of modern life.

Physical activity isn't just a way to burn calories or sculpt muscles; it's a fundamental pillar of cardiovascular resilience. When we move, our hearts grow stronger, our blood vessels become more flexible, and our entire circulatory system operates with a efficiency that no synthetic drug can replicate. Regular exercise improves circulation by enhancing the ability of blood vessels to expand and contract, a process called endothelial function. This means nutrients and oxygen reach our tissues more effectively, while waste products are cleared away before they can cause damage. Studies have consistently shown that even moderate activity -- like brisk walking or gardening -- can lower blood pressure as effectively as some medications, without the side effects or long-term dependencies. And unlike pharmaceuticals, which often mask symptoms while ignoring root causes, exercise addresses the underlying imbalances that lead to heart disease in the first place.

Not all movement is created equal, though, and understanding the unique benefits of different types of exercise can help you tailor a routine that truly supports your heart. Aerobic exercises, like jogging, swimming, or cycling, are the cornerstone of cardiovascular endurance. They train your heart to pump blood more efficiently, reducing the strain on your arteries and lowering resting heart rate -- a key marker of long-term heart health. But strength training plays an equally critical role. Lifting weights, resistance band work, or even bodyweight exercises like squats and push-ups don't just build muscle; they improve metabolic health by increasing insulin sensitivity, which helps regulate blood sugar and reduces inflammation. This is crucial because chronic inflammation and insulin resistance are silent drivers of heart disease, often overlooked by conventional medicine. Meanwhile, practices like yoga and tai chi, which blend movement with breath control, have been shown to reduce stress hormones like cortisol, which can otherwise damage blood vessels over time.

One of the most overlooked yet profound benefits of exercise is its ability to combat inflammation and support weight management -- two of the biggest threats to heart health in today's world. Chronic inflammation isn't just a byproduct of poor diet or environmental toxins; it's also fueled by inactivity. When muscles contract during exercise, they release anti-inflammatory molecules that help neutralize the damage caused by processed foods, electromagnetic pollution, and even emotional stress. At the same time, physical activity directly improves insulin sensitivity, allowing your body to use glucose more effectively instead of storing it as fat. This dual action -- reducing inflammation while optimizing metabolism -- creates a protective shield around your heart, lowering the risk of plaque buildup in arteries and preventing the metabolic syndrome that so often leads to heart attacks and strokes.

But the benefits of exercise go even deeper, down to the cellular level. Every time you engage in physical activity, your body ramps up production of mitochondria --the tiny powerhouses inside your cells that generate energy. More mitochondria mean more efficient energy production, which translates to better endurance, faster recovery, and a heart that can handle stress without faltering. Exercise also triggers autophagy, a natural process where your cells clean out damaged components and recycle them into new, healthier structures. This cellular "housekeeping" is critical for preventing the oxidative damage that accelerates aging and weakens the cardiovascular system. In essence, movement doesn't just keep your heart beating -- it helps your cells repair themselves, ensuring your entire body stays resilient against the wear and tear of modern life.

So how do you harness these benefits in a way that's sustainable and effective? The key lies in consistency, progression, and listening to your body. You don't need to run marathons or spend hours in the gym to protect your heart. Research suggests that as little as 150 minutes of moderate-intensity exercise per week --about 20 minutes a day -- can significantly reduce the risk of heart disease. This could be a combination of brisk walking, cycling, or even dancing in your living room. The important thing is to move regularly, allowing your body to adapt gradually. Start with what feels manageable, then slowly increase the intensity or duration as your fitness improves. For example, if walking is your baseline, try adding short bursts of faster pacing (interval training to challenge your heart in new ways. Strength training should be incorporated at least twice a week, focusing on compound movements that engage multiple muscle groups, like deadlifts or lunges. And don't underestimate the power of everyday movement --taking the stairs, gardening, or playing with your kids all contribute to a heart-healthy lifestyle.

Of course, life isn't always cooperative, and barriers like time constraints, lack of motivation, or physical limitations can make exercise feel out of reach. But these challenges aren't insurmountable -- they're opportunities to get creative. If time is an issue, break your workouts into shorter segments: three 10-minute walks spread throughout the day can be just as effective as a single 30-minute session. Struggling with motivation? Find an activity you genuinely enjoy, whether it's hiking in nature, joining a local sports league, or following along with a home

workout video. The more pleasure you associate with movement, the easier it becomes to stick with it. For those with physical limitations, low-impact options like swimming, water aerobics, or chair yoga can provide tremendous benefits without straining joints or exacerbating injuries. The goal isn't perfection; it's progress. Every step you take, no matter how small, is a step toward a stronger heart.

It's also important to recognize that more isn't always better. In a culture that often glorifies extreme fitness, it's easy to fall into the trap of overtraining, which can backfire by increasing stress hormones, suppressing immune function, and even damaging the heart over time. Signs of overtraining include persistent fatigue, elevated resting heart rate, insomnia, and frequent illnesses -- all red flags that your body needs rest. Recovery is just as critical as the exercise itself, giving your heart and muscles time to repair and grow stronger. Incorporate rest days into your routine, prioritize sleep, and consider practices like meditation or deep breathing to lower stress levels. Remember, the goal is resilience, not exhaustion.

Consider the story of Mark, a 52-year-old office worker who came to me after a routine checkup revealed high blood pressure and borderline diabetes. His doctor had prescribed statins and blood pressure medication, but Mark was skeptical.

He'd watched his father suffer through years of pharmaceutical side effects, only to die of a heart attack at 65. Instead of filling the prescriptions, Mark committed to a structured exercise program:

three days of brisk walking, two days of strength training, and weekend hikes with his family. Within three months, his blood pressure dropped to normal levels, his blood sugar stabilized, and he'd lost 15 pounds -- without a single pill. More importantly, he felt stronger, more energetic, and more in control of his health than he had in years. His story isn't unique; it's a testament to what the body can achieve when given the chance to heal naturally.

The takeaway is clear: your heart wasn't designed to thrive in a world of sedentary convenience, processed foods, and pharmaceutical quick fixes. It was designed to move, to adapt, and to heal. In a system that profits from sickness, exercise is one of the last true acts of self-reliance -- a way to reclaim your health without relying on institutions that have repeatedly failed us. Whether you're just starting out or looking to deepen your routine, remember that every movement counts. Your heart doesn't care if you're in a gym or your backyard, lifting weights or carrying groceries. What matters is that you keep moving, keep challenging yourself, and trust in your body's innate ability to heal. In a world that's increasingly toxic --physically, emotionally, and spiritually -- physical activity is more than just a habit. It's an act of resistance, a declaration of independence, and one of the most powerful tools you have to live a long, vibrant, and free life.

Reducing Toxic Load to Improve Heart Function Naturally

Imagine your body as a finely tuned engine -- one that thrives when given clean fuel, fresh air, and proper maintenance. But what happens when that engine is clogged with sludge, rust, and debris? It sputters, struggles, and eventually breaks down. The same is true for your heart. Every day, your body is bombarded with invisible toxins from the air you breathe, the food you eat, and the products you use. Over time, these toxins build up, creating what's known as toxic load -- a silent burden that strains your heart and accelerates disease.

The good news? You don't need expensive drugs or risky procedures to turn things around. By reducing your toxic load naturally, you can restore your heart's vitality, improve circulation, and reclaim your health -- all while sidestepping the harmful interventions pushed by a corrupt medical system that profits from sickness.

Toxic load isn't just a buzzword; it's the cumulative effect of years -- or even decades -- of exposure to harmful substances that your body wasn't designed to handle. These toxins come from everywhere: the pesticide residues on conventionally grown produce, the heavy metals like mercury in dental fillings or contaminated fish, the microplastics leaching from water bottles and food packaging, and the industrial chemicals lurking in household cleaners and personal care products. Even the air you breathe, especially in urban areas, carries a cocktail of pollutants from vehicle exhaust, factory emissions, and the toxic fallout of geoengineering programs like chemtrails. Your body does its best to filter and eliminate these invaders, but when the load becomes too great, toxins get stored in fat tissues, lodge in arteries, and disrupt the delicate balance of your cells. Over time, this buildup doesn't just wear you down -- it actively sabotages your heart by triggering inflammation, oxidizing your arteries, and impairing the endothelial cells that line your blood vessels.

The cardiovascular risks of these toxins are staggering -- and deliberately downplayed by a medical establishment that would rather prescribe statins than address the root cause. Heavy metals like lead and cadmium, for example, are strongly linked to hypertension and atherosclerosis because they damage the endothelial lining of your blood vessels, making them stiff and prone to plaque buildup. Pesticides like glyphosate, the active ingredient in Roundup, don't just kill weeds; they disrupt your gut microbiome, impair mitochondrial function, and contribute to chronic inflammation -- a key driver of heart disease. Then there are the endocrine-disrupting chemicals in plastics, such as BPA and phthalates, which mimic hormones and throw your metabolic health into chaos, increasing your risk of obesity, diabetes, and heart failure. And let's not forget the airborne pollutants like fine particulate matter (PM2.5), which studies show can trigger heart attacks and strokes by causing oxidative stress and reducing blood flow. These aren't just theoretical risks -- they're real, measurable threats that Big Pharma and regulatory agencies like the FDA and EPA have failed to protect you from, often because they're in bed with the very industries poisoning you.

So how exactly do these toxins wreak havoc on your heart? The answer lies in three interconnected processes: oxidative stress, inflammation, and endothelial dysfunction. Oxidative stress occurs when toxins generate an excess of free radicals -- unstable molecules that attack your cells, damaging DNA, proteins, and lipids. Your heart, with its high demand for energy, is particularly vulnerable.

Chronic inflammation follows, as your immune system remains in a constant state of alert, releasing pro-inflammatory cytokines that thicken arterial walls and promote clot formation. Meanwhile, endothelial dysfunction -- the inability of your blood vessels to dilate properly -- sets the stage for hypertension and atherosclerosis. This trifecta doesn't just contribute to heart disease; it accelerates it, turning what could be a manageable condition into a life-threatening crisis. The tragedy? Most doctors will never tell you this because they're trained to treat symptoms, not causes -- and because the real solutions don't involve patented drugs.

The path to a healthier heart begins with reducing your toxic load, and the most powerful tool you have is your diet. Start by eliminating processed foods, which are laced with artificial additives, refined sugars, and industrial seed oils that fuel inflammation and oxidative damage. Instead, focus on organic, whole foods --especially those rich in antioxidants, like berries, leafy greens, and cruciferous vegetables, which help neutralize free radicals. Incorporate foods that bind and escort toxins out of your body, such as cilantro and chlorella for heavy metals, and ground flaxseeds for excess estrogen and xenoestrogens. Grass-fed meats and wild-caught fish (from low-mercury sources provide clean protein without the hormonal disruptors found in factory-farmed animals. And don't forget filtered water -- reverse osmosis or activated carbon filters can remove heavy metals, fluoride, and microplastics that municipal water systems often leave behind. Your kitchen should be a sanctuary, not a source of toxicity.

But diet is just one piece of the puzzle. The air you breathe and the water you drink are just as critical. Indoor air can be even more polluted than outdoor air, thanks to off-gassing from furniture, synthetic carpets, and cleaning products. Invest in a high-quality HEPA air purifier to capture fine particles, and consider adding houseplants like snake plants or peace lilies, which naturally filter common toxins like benzene and formaldehyde. For water, avoid plastic bottles at all costs --opt for glass or stainless steel containers, and if you're on municipal water, test for contaminants like lead, chlorine, and PFAS (the "forever chemicals" found in non-stick cookware and firefighting foam). Even your personal care routine matters: swap out conventional shampoos, deodorants, and lotions for natural alternatives free of parabens, sulfates, and synthetic fragrances. Your skin is your largest organ, and what you put on it ends up in your bloodstream -- and eventually, your heart.

Your body is equipped with its own detoxification systems -- the liver, kidneys, lymphatic system, and even your skin -- but these pathways need support to function optimally. The liver, your primary detox organ, relies on nutrients like milk thistle, NAC (N-acetylcysteine, and B vitamins to process and eliminate toxins.

Your kidneys filter waste from your blood, but they need adequate hydration and electrolytes to do their job. The lymphatic system, often overlooked, depends on movement -- rebounding on a mini trampoline or dry brushing your skin can stimulate lymph flow and help clear stagnant toxins. And then there's your skin, which eliminates waste through sweat. This is where practices like infrared sauna therapy shine: by inducing a deep, detoxifying sweat, saunas help remove heavy metals, pesticides, and even plastic residues while improving circulation and reducing blood pressure. Castor oil packs, applied to the abdomen, can enhance lymphatic drainage and liver function, offering a gentle yet effective way to support your body's natural cleansing processes.

For those who think detoxification requires extreme juice fasts or expensive clinics, think again. The most effective strategies are simple, time-tested, and rooted in natural medicine -- practices that have been suppressed by a medical industry that profits from keeping you sick. Sauna therapy, for example, isn't just relaxing; it's a scientifically proven way to reduce toxic load. Studies show that regular sauna use can lower levels of heavy metals like lead and mercury while improving endothelial function and reducing the risk of cardiovascular events. Dry brushing, a technique that involves brushing your skin with a natural bristle brush before showering, stimulates lymphatic drainage and helps your body eliminate waste more efficiently. Castor oil packs, another underrated remedy, draw toxins out of tissues while reducing inflammation -- a double win for heart health. Even something as simple as deep breathing exercises can enhance oxygenation and support your body's detox pathways. These aren't fads; they're tools for reclaiming your health in a world that's increasingly toxic.

Let's talk about a real-life example: a 58-year-old man named Mark who came to me with high blood pressure, fatigue, and a family history of heart disease. His doctor had him on three medications, yet his symptoms were worsening. After testing, we discovered elevated levels of lead, arsenic, and glyphosate in his system -- likely from years of eating conventional foods, drinking unfiltered tap water, and living near a busy highway. Instead of adding more pills, we focused on reducing his toxic load. Mark switched to an organic, anti-inflammatory diet, installed a whole-house water filter, and started using an infrared sauna three times a week. He replaced his synthetic deodorant and laundry detergent with natural alternatives and began taking binders like activated charcoal and zeolite to help pull heavy metals from his tissues. Within three months, his blood pressure normalized, his energy returned, and his follow-up tests showed a significant drop in toxin levels. His doctor was stunned -- and, predictably, tried to take credit for the "spontaneous improvement." But Mark knew the truth: his body had been drowning in toxins, and once he gave it the tools to cleanse, it healed itself.

The biggest myth about detoxification is that it's only for "cleanses" or extreme protocols. In reality, detox is a daily process -- one that your body is designed to handle, provided you give it the right support. You don't need to live in a bubble or spend a fortune on supplements to reduce your toxic load. Start small: swap one processed food for an organic alternative, drink filtered water, and open your windows to freshen the air in your home. Gradually, these changes add up, reducing the burden on your heart and allowing your body to function as it was meant to. Remember, the goal isn't perfection -- it's progress. Every toxin you avoid, every natural choice you make, is a step toward a stronger, healthier heart. And in a world where the medical system is more interested in managing disease than preventing it, taking control of your toxic load isn't just smart -- it's an act of rebellion against a system that wants to keep you dependent, sick, and compliant. Your heart deserves better. And with the right knowledge and tools, you can give it exactly that.

The Importance of Quality Sleep for Heart Disease Prevention

In a world where our health is constantly under siege by processed foods, environmental toxins, and the stress of modern living, it's more important than ever to take control of our well-being. One of the most powerful, yet often overlooked, tools in our natural health arsenal is quality sleep. In this section, we'll explore the profound impact that sleep has on our heart health and provide you with practical, natural strategies to improve your sleep and, in turn, your cardiovascular well-being.

During sleep, our bodies undergo a remarkable process of repair and rejuvenation. It's a time when our blood pressure naturally dips, giving our hearts a much-needed rest. This nightly dip in blood pressure is crucial for maintaining a healthy cardiovascular system. Moreover, sleep is when our bodies repair damaged tissues, including those in our blood vessels, helping to prevent the buildup of plaque that can lead to heart disease. Sleep also plays a vital role in regulating our metabolism and reducing inflammation, both of which are key factors in maintaining heart health.

Poor sleep, on the other hand, has been linked to a host of cardiovascular problems. Chronic sleep deprivation can lead to consistently elevated blood pressure, increasing the risk of hypertension, heart disease, and stroke. When we don't get enough sleep, our bodies produce more stress hormones, which can cause inflammation and damage to our blood vessels. Furthermore, poor sleep disrupts our circadian rhythms, the natural cycles that govern our bodily functions. These disruptions can lead to imbalances in our hormones, metabolism, and immune function, all of which can negatively impact our heart health.

The good news is that there are many natural, effective ways to improve our sleep quality. One of the most important is maintaining good sleep hygiene. This includes going to bed and waking up at the same time each day, even on weekends. It also means creating a sleep-friendly environment in your bedroom: keep it cool, dark, and quiet, and reserve it for sleep and intimacy only. Avoid screens for at least an hour before bed, as the blue light they emit can interfere with your body's production of melatonin, a hormone that regulates sleep.

Certain nutrients and herbs can also support healthy sleep. Magnesium, for instance, is a mineral that plays a crucial role in regulating our sleep cycles. It can be found in foods like leafy greens, nuts, and seeds, or taken as a supplement.

Valerian root is another natural sleep aid that has been used for centuries. It can help to reduce the time it takes to fall asleep and improve sleep quality. Melatonin supplements can also be helpful, especially for those who have trouble falling asleep or who do shift work.

Common sleep disorders, such as insomnia and sleep apnea, can significantly impact our heart health. Insomnia, characterized by difficulty falling or staying asleep, can lead to chronic sleep deprivation and its associated cardiovascular risks. Sleep apnea, a condition where breathing repeatedly stops and starts during sleep, can cause sudden drops in blood pressure and oxygen levels, putting a strain on the heart. If you suspect you have a sleep disorder, it's important to seek help from a healthcare provider who is knowledgeable about natural, non-pharmaceutical treatments.

Consistency in our sleep patterns is also vital for heart health. Our bodies thrive on routine, and going to bed and waking up at the same time each day helps to regulate our circadian rhythms. Shift work or irregular sleep schedules can disrupt these rhythms, leading to a host of health problems, including an increased risk of heart disease. If you do shift work, it's especially important to prioritize sleep and create a dark, quiet sleep environment during the day.

Let's consider the case of John, a 45-year-old man who was struggling with high blood pressure and poor sleep. John worked long hours at a stressful job and often stayed up late watching TV. He would wake up feeling exhausted and rely on coffee to get through the day. After learning about the importance of sleep for heart health, John made some changes. He started going to bed and waking up at the same time each day, even on weekends. He created a relaxing bedtime routine that included reading and a warm bath. He also started taking a magnesium supplement and drinking chamomile tea before bed. Within a few weeks, John noticed a significant improvement in his sleep quality. He felt more rested during the day and, over time, his blood pressure began to normalize.

Improving our sleep is one of the most powerful, natural strategies we have for preventing heart disease. By understanding the profound impact that sleep has on our cardiovascular health and making simple, natural changes to improve our sleep quality, we can take a significant step towards optimal heart health.

Remember, our bodies have an incredible capacity for healing and regeneration when given the right tools and environment. Prioritizing sleep is one of the best ways we can support our bodies' natural healing processes and maintain our heart health.

In our journey towards optimal heart health, it's crucial to remember that we are not just physical beings, but spiritual ones as well. Our consciousness, our spirit, plays a vital role in our overall well-being. As we prioritize sleep and make other natural, healthful changes in our lives, let's also nurture our spiritual health. This can be as simple as taking a few moments each day for quiet reflection, prayer, or meditation. By caring for our bodies, minds, and spirits, we can truly thrive and live our lives to the fullest.

Managing Stress Through Mindfulness, Breathwork, and Meditation

Stress isn't just that tight feeling in your shoulders or the racing thoughts that keep you up at night -- it's a silent saboteur, quietly wreaking havoc on your heart. When you're stressed, your body reacts as if you're facing a physical threat, even if the danger is just an overflowing inbox or a traffic jam. Your adrenal glands pump out cortisol, your heart rate spikes, and your blood vessels constrict. Over time, this chronic stress response -- governed by the hypothalamic-pituitary-adrenal (HPA) axis and the sympathetic nervous system -- becomes a one-way ticket to inflammation, high blood pressure, and even heart disease. The medical establishment might push pills to mask the symptoms, but the real solution lies in reclaiming control of your nervous system through time-tested, natural practices: mindfulness, breathwork, and meditation.

These aren't just feel-good buzzwords; they're powerful tools backed by science. Mindfulness, for instance, trains your brain to stay present instead of spiraling into anxiety about the future or regret about the past. Studies show that regular mindfulness practice can lower cortisol levels, reduce systemic inflammation, and even improve heart rate variability (HRV) -- a key marker of cardiovascular resilience. When your HRV is high, your heart can adapt more flexibly to stress, which means less wear and tear on your arteries and a lower risk of conditions like hypertension or Takotsubo cardiomyopathy, a stress-induced heart syndrome that mimics a heart attack. The beauty of mindfulness is that it doesn't require a prescription or a doctor's approval -- just your attention and a willingness to pause.

Then there's breathwork, a practice so simple yet so profound that it can shift your physiology in minutes. Diaphragmatic breathing -- where you breathe deeply into your belly rather than shallowly into your chest -- activates your parasympathetic nervous system, the body's built-in 'rest and digest' mode. This counters the fight-or-flight response, lowering blood pressure and reducing the strain on your heart. Research published in Human Heart, Cosmic Heart by Dr. Thomas Cowan highlights how controlled breathing techniques can improve oxygenation and circulation, which are critical for heart health. Even loving-kindness meditation, where you focus on sending compassion to yourself and others, has been shown to reduce arterial stiffness, a risk factor for atherosclerosis. These practices don't just calm your mind; they literally reshape your cardiovascular system for the better.

But how do these practices actually work on a biological level? Let's break it down. When you meditate or engage in slow, deliberate breathing, your brain releases neurotransmitters like GABA, which act as natural tranquilizers, easing the hyperactivity of your stress response. At the same time, your body reduces the production of inflammatory cytokines -- molecules that, when chronically elevated, damage the endothelial lining of your blood vessels and set the stage for plaque buildup. A study referenced in The Science of Pain Is Changing Rapidly on Mercola.com underscores how mindfulness can modulate pain perception and inflammation, which are closely linked to cardiovascular health. Meanwhile, techniques like body scan meditation -- where you mentally scan your body for tension and release it -- help dissolve physical stress patterns that contribute to hypertension.

If you're new to these practices, start small. Even five minutes a day of diaphragmatic breathing can make a difference. Sit or lie down, place one hand on your belly, and inhale deeply through your nose for four counts, letting your abdomen expand. Exhale slowly for six counts, feeling your belly deflate. Repeat.

For mindfulness, try anchoring yourself in the present by focusing on your senses: the feel of your feet on the ground, the sound of your breath, the taste of your tea. Apps like Insight Timer or simple guided meditations on YouTube can help if you're struggling to quiet your mind. Advanced practitioners might explore longer sits or breathwork techniques like the Wim Hof Method, which combines breathing exercises with cold exposure to supercharge stress resilience.

One of the biggest barriers people face is the myth that they 'don't have time' for these practices. But here's the truth: you don't have time not to do them. Chronic stress isn't just a mental burden -- it's a physiological emergency that accelerates aging, weakens your immune system, and strains your heart. The good news? You can weave mindfulness and breathwork into your daily routine without adding extra time. Try mindful eating -- savoring each bite without distraction -- or practice box breathing (four counts in, four counts hold, four counts out, four counts hold while stuck in traffic. Even a one-minute pause to focus on your breath before a meeting can reset your nervous system.

These practices become even more powerful when combined with other natural stress-busters like exercise, sunlight, and social connection. Movement, especially outdoors, enhances the effects of meditation by boosting endorphins and grounding your body in nature's rhythms. Meanwhile, strong social ties -- whether through family, friends, or community -- buffer against stress by providing emotional support and reducing feelings of isolation. The corporate medical system wants you to believe that heart health is all about cholesterol numbers and prescription drugs, but the real medicine is in how you live: how you breathe, how you think, and how you connect with the world around you.

Consider the case of Mark, a 52-year-old executive who came to me after a stress-induced cardiac event. His doctors put him on beta-blockers and told him to 'reduce stress,' but they offered no real tools to do so. Mark started with just ten minutes of mindfulness meditation each morning, paired with diaphragmatic breathing exercises during his commute. Within three months, his blood pressure dropped from 150/95 to 125/80, his HRV improved by 30%, and his need for medication decreased. More importantly, he reported feeling 'lighter,' both emotionally and physically. His story isn't unique -- it's a testament to the body's innate capacity to heal when given the right conditions. The pharmaceutical industry may profit from keeping you dependent on pills, but your heart thrives on the simplicity of your breath, the stillness of your mind, and the warmth of human connection.

The road to heart health isn't paved with statins or surgical interventions; it's built on daily choices that honor your body's wisdom. Mindfulness, breathwork, and meditation aren't just complementary therapies -- they're foundational pillars of a life free from the grip of chronic stress. In a world that profits from your fear and fatigue, these practices are acts of rebellion, reclaiming your power to heal. Start today. Breathe deeply. Stay present. Your heart will thank you.

REFERENCES:

- *Cowan, Thomas. Human Heart, Cosmic Heart: A Doctor's Quest to Understand, Treat, and Prevent Cardiovascular Disease*

- *Mercola.com. The Science of Pain Is Changing Rapidly*

Building Social Connections to Support Long-Term Heart Health

There's a quiet epidemic sweeping across modern society -- one that doesn't make headlines like the latest pharmaceutical breakthrough or government health mandate. It's not a virus, a toxin, or a genetic flaw. It's loneliness. And its toll on heart health is just as real as smoking, poor diet, or a sedentary lifestyle. Decades of research, much of it buried under the noise of Big Pharma's drug-pushing campaigns, reveal something profound: the strength of our social bonds may be the most underrated tool we have for preventing -- and even reversing -- heart disease. This isn't just feel-good advice; it's biology. Our bodies are wired to thrive in connection, and when that connection is missing, the damage shows up in our arteries, our blood pressure, and even our survival rates after a heart attack.

At the core of this connection is oxytocin, often called the 'love hormone,' though it's far more than that. Oxytocin is released when we hug a friend, laugh with family, or even pet a dog. It acts like a natural beta-blocker, lowering stress hormones like cortisol and adrenaline that, when chronically elevated, inflame our blood vessels and strain our hearts. Studies on tribal societies -- where people live in tight-knit communities -- show remarkably low rates of heart disease, not because they have access to statins or stents, but because their daily lives are woven with social rituals, shared meals, and mutual support. Compare that to the modern Western lifestyle, where people eat alone in front of screens, communicate in text bubbles, and outsource their healthcare to a system that profits from their sickness. The contrast isn't just sad -- it's deadly. Chronic loneliness has been linked to a 29% increased risk of heart disease and a 32% higher risk of stroke, rivaling the dangers of obesity or high blood pressure. And unlike those conditions, loneliness doesn't require a prescription to fix. It requires something far simpler: other people.

But here's where the story gets even more disturbing. Loneliness doesn't just make us feel bad -- it rewires our bodies for disease. When we're isolated, our immune systems go haywire, producing more inflammatory cytokines, the same molecules that damage arterial walls and set the stage for plaque buildup. Our sleep suffers, our blood pressure creeps up, and we're more likely to self-soothe with processed foods, alcohol, or hours of mindless scrolling -- all of which feed the fire of cardiovascular decline. Worse, isolated individuals are less likely to seek help when symptoms arise, often because they lack someone to notice the warning signs. This isn't speculation; it's documented in studies like the one from Social Science & Medicine, which found that socially isolated men had a 90% higher risk of cardiovascular death than those with strong social ties. Meanwhile, women with robust friendships were shown to produce more oxytocin during stress, effectively buffering their hearts from damage. The message is clear: our relationships aren't just a side dish to health -- they're the main course.

Now, consider what happens when those relationships are strong. After a heart attack, patients with high levels of social support are three times more likely to survive the first year compared to those who are alone. That's not because their doctors are better or their medications stronger -- it's because they have people who remind them to take their herbs, join them for walks, and offer a reason to keep fighting. In Blue Zones -- regions where people live the longest, healthiest lives -- centenarians don't just eat well and move naturally; they belong to tight-knit communities where elders are revered, meals are shared, and purpose is collective. Their 'medicine' isn't a pill; it's a potluck. And the data backs this up: a meta-analysis in PLOS Medicine found that people with strong social ties had a 50% higher likelihood of survival over time, regardless of their initial health status. That's a bigger impact than quitting smoking. Yet how many cardiologists write prescriptions for 'one dinner party per week' or 'daily phone calls with a loved one'? The system isn't designed to heal -- it's designed to bill.

The good news is that building these connections doesn't require a village elder or a perfect family. It starts with small, intentional choices. Join a gardening club where you can swap homegrown veggies and recipes for heart-healthy meals.

Volunteer at an animal shelter -- studies show that petting a dog for just 15 minutes lowers cortisol and boosts oxytocin, and dog owners have a 24% lower risk of death from heart disease. Host a weekly potluck where the rule is 'no processed foods allowed,' turning nutrition into a shared adventure. Even virtual communities, when built around shared values like natural health or preparedness, can provide meaningful support -- though they're no substitute for in-person connection. The key is consistency. Our bodies respond to repeated doses of connection, just like they respond to repeated doses of a toxin. One lonely weekend won't kill you, but a life of isolation will.

Of course, there are barriers. The same system that profits from sickness also profits from keeping us too busy, too distracted, and too divided to form real bonds. Social media, for all its promises of connection, often leaves us more isolated, comparing our lives to curated highlight reels while our oxytocin levels plummet. Busy schedules, long commutes, and the erosion of third spaces -- like churches, community centers, and local markets -- make it harder to bump into neighbors, let alone form deep friendships. And for those who've been hurt by toxic relationships, the idea of 'putting yourself out there' can feel risky. But here's the truth: quality matters more than quantity. A single trusted friend who shares your values -- whether it's growing your own food, questioning mainstream narratives, or prioritizing natural health -- can be more protective than a dozen shallow acquaintances. Conversely, a stressful or manipulative relationship can spike your cortisol as much as a fast-food meal. The goal isn't to collect contacts; it's to cultivate allies.

Take the case of Mark, a 58-year-old man who came to me after a mild heart attack. His doctor had put him on statins and blood pressure meds, but his real problem wasn't cholesterol -- it was isolation. Divorced, retired, and living in a suburb where no one knew his name, he'd spent years eating microwave dinners in front of the news, his only social interaction the cashier at the pharmacy. We didn't just tweak his diet (though we cut out processed foods); we built a plan to rebuild his community. He started volunteering at a local farm co-op, trading his accounting skills for fresh produce. He joined a men's hiking group that met weekly in the mountains. Within six months, his blood pressure dropped enough to reduce his medication, his inflammatory markers improved, and -- perhaps most telling -- he laughed more. His 'treatment' wasn't a drug; it was a life. And that's the power of connection: it doesn't just add years to your life; it adds life to your years.

For those who feel stuck, start small. If joining a club feels overwhelming, strike up a conversation with the person next to you at the farmers' market. If you're introverted, try one-on-one activities like trading homegrown herbs with a neighbor or joining a book club focused on natural health. If time is the issue, combine socializing with movement -- walking meetings, dance classes, or even a weekly 'weeding party' in your garden. And if you've been burned by toxic relationships in the past, remember: healthy connections are built on mutual respect, not obligation. You don't owe anyone your energy, but you do owe it to yourself to seek out people who align with your values -- whether that's sovereignty, preparedness, or simply the joy of a shared meal.

The final piece of the puzzle? Recognize that this isn't just about you. When you strengthen your social ties, you're not just protecting your heart -- you're creating a ripple effect. Your oxytocin-fueled calm can lower stress for those around you. Your shared meals become a model for others to break free from processed foods. Your community garden becomes a hub for bartering skills and knowledge, reducing reliance on corrupt systems. In a world where institutions profit from division -- whether it's Big Pharma selling antidepressants for loneliness or governments using isolation to control populations -- choosing connection is an act of rebellion. It's a way to opt out of the sickness industry and into a life of real health, built on the oldest medicine of all: each other.

So here's your prescription, no insurance required: Reach out. Show up. Let people in. Your heart -- literally -- depends on it.

Avoiding Common Dietary Pitfalls That Harm Cardiovascular Function

The modern food landscape is a minefield of hidden dangers, carefully engineered to keep you hooked while quietly destroying your heart. For decades, centralized institutions -- government agencies, Big Food corporations, and their allies in mainstream medicine -- have pushed a diet that lines their pockets while sabotaging your health. The truth is, most chronic heart disease isn't an inevitable part of aging -- it's the direct result of daily dietary choices that trigger inflammation, metabolic chaos, and arterial damage. But here's the good news: by recognizing and avoiding these common pitfalls, you can reclaim control of your cardiovascular destiny.

Let's start with the most insidious culprit: refined sugar and its close cousin, refined carbohydrates. These aren't just empty calories -- they're metabolic poisons. When you consume sugary drinks, pastries, or even 'healthy' whole-grain breads made from refined flour, your blood sugar spikes dramatically. This forces your pancreas to pump out insulin, the hormone that tells your cells to absorb glucose. Over time, this constant barrage of sugar and insulin leads to insulin resistance, where your cells essentially 'tune out' the signal. The result? Your body stores more fat, your triglycerides skyrocket, and inflammation rages through your arteries like a wildfire. Studies confirm that high sugar intake directly accelerates atherosclerosis -- the hardening and narrowing of arteries -- that sets the stage for heart attacks and strokes. And don't be fooled by 'natural' sugars like agave or honey; while slightly better than high-fructose corn syrup, they still contribute to the same metabolic dysfunction when consumed in excess.

Then there's the myth of 'heart-healthy' vegetable oils -- a lie perpetuated by the same industries that profit from selling them. Soybean oil, corn oil, canola oil, and other processed vegetable oils are anything but healthy. These oils are chemically unstable and prone to oxidation, which means they generate free radicals that damage your endothelial cells -- the delicate lining of your blood vessels. Worse, they're loaded with omega-6 fatty acids, which, when consumed in excess without balancing omega-3s, fuel chronic inflammation. This isn't just theory; research shows that populations consuming high amounts of these oils have significantly higher rates of coronary artery disease. The food industry loves them because they're cheap and extend shelf life, but your heart pays the price. Even 'trans fat-free' labels are deceptive -- many processed foods still contain partially hydrogenated oils, which behave like trans fats in your body, stiffening your arteries and increasing your risk of sudden cardiac death.

Processed foods are another silent killer, disguised as convenience. That frozen dinner, deli meat, or bag of chips isn't just lacking in nutrients -- it's packed with sodium, artificial preservatives, and flavor enhancers like MSG that overstimulate your nervous system and disrupt your metabolism. Excess sodium doesn't just raise your blood pressure; it alters the delicate balance of minerals in your body, forcing your heart to work harder while your kidneys struggle to keep up. And let's not forget the artificial additives -- many of which have never been properly tested for long-term safety. These chemicals don't just sit inertly in your body; they interact with your gut microbiome, your immune system, and your vascular function in ways we're only beginning to understand. The solution isn't to trust 'low-fat' or 'diet' labels -- those are often the worst offenders, replacing fat with sugar and synthetic fillers that leave you hungrier and sicker.

Alcohol is another dietary pitfall that's often glorified in our culture, but the truth is far less glamorous. While a glass of red wine now and then might have some cardiovascular benefits thanks to resveratrol, regular or heavy drinking is a one-way ticket to heart damage. Alcohol is a toxin that your liver has to detoxify, and in the process, it raises your blood pressure, weakens your heart muscle (a condition called cardiomyopathy, and disrupts your heart's electrical rhythms. Over time, it also depletes critical nutrients like magnesium and B vitamins, which are essential for maintaining healthy blood vessels and preventing arrhythmias. The idea that 'moderate' drinking is harmless is a myth pushed by an industry that profits from addiction. Your heart doesn't care about cultural norms -- it only responds to the biochemical stress you put on it.

So how do you navigate this toxic food environment? Start by taking back control of your kitchen. Cooking from scratch with whole, unprocessed ingredients isn't just a health strategy -- it's an act of rebellion against a system that wants to keep you dependent on their poisonous products. Learn to read labels like a detective: if you can't pronounce an ingredient or it sounds like it belongs in a chemistry lab, put it back. Focus on foods in their natural state -- grass-fed meats, wild-caught fish, organic vegetables, nuts, seeds, and fruits. These foods don't just avoid harm; they actively heal. For example, the omega-3s in fatty fish like salmon reduce inflammation, while the antioxidants in berries protect your endothelial cells from oxidative damage. And don't fear healthy fats -- avocados, olive oil, coconut oil, and butter from grass-fed cows are your heart's allies, not enemies. The low-fat craze was a lie designed to sell processed junk food, and it's time to reject it.

Mindful eating is another powerful tool. In a world that encourages mindless consumption -- eating in front of screens, rushing through meals, ignoring hunger cues -- reconnecting with your body's natural signals can transform your health.

Your body knows when it's hungry and when it's full, but years of processed food addiction have dulled those signals. Start by eating slowly, chewing thoroughly, and paying attention to the flavors and textures of your food. This not only improves digestion but also helps you recognize true satiety, preventing overeating. And remember: hunger isn't an emergency. It's okay to feel a little hungry between meals -- it gives your body a chance to burn fat and repair itself. Intermittent fasting, where you extend the overnight fast by skipping breakfast or eating an early dinner, is one of the most effective ways to improve insulin sensitivity and reduce cardiovascular risk.

One of the biggest myths you'll hear is that all fats are bad for your heart. This is a deliberate deception meant to keep you buying low-fat, high-sugar products that make food corporations rich while making you sick. The truth is, your heart needs healthy fats to function. Your cell membranes, including those in your heart and blood vessels, are made of fats. Your brain -- which controls your heart rate and blood pressure -- is 60% fat. The key is choosing the right fats: saturated fats from animal sources (yes, even butter and lard, monounsaturated fats like olive oil, and omega-3s from fish and flaxseeds. These fats reduce inflammation, stabilize your heart's electrical activity, and provide steady energy without the blood sugar rollercoaster. The fats to avoid are the processed, oxidized ones found in fried foods, margarine, and packaged snacks. Nature didn't design those -- corporate labs did.

Let me tell you about James, a 58-year-old man who came to me after suffering a minor heart attack. His doctors put him on statins, blood pressure meds, and a low-fat diet, but his energy was still terrible, and his cholesterol numbers weren't improving. When we dug into his diet, we found he was eating 'heart-healthy' cereal for breakfast, a turkey sandwich on whole wheat for lunch, and lean chicken with pasta for dinner -- all washed down with diet soda. In other words, he was consuming a steady stream of refined carbs, processed meats, and artificial sweeteners. We switched him to a diet rich in healthy fats, pasture-raised eggs, wild salmon, and plenty of vegetables. Within three months, his triglycerides dropped by 60%, his blood pressure normalized, and he had enough energy to start exercising again. A year later, his doctor was stunned -- his coronary calcium score, a measure of plaque in his arteries, had actually decreased. James didn't just avoid another heart attack; he reversed the damage. His story isn't unique --it's what happens when you stop feeding your body poison and start giving it what it truly needs.

The path to a healthy heart isn't about deprivation -- it's about liberation. Liberation from the lies of the food industry, the pharmaceutical complex, and the government agencies that serve them. It's about reclaiming your right to eat real, nourishing food that heals rather than harms. Every time you choose an avocado over a bag of chips, cook a meal from scratch instead of microwaving a frozen dinner, or skip the dessert tray at a restaurant, you're not just making a health choice -- you're casting a vote for a world where people, not corporations, control their own well-being. Your heart is resilient, designed to beat strongly for decades if given the right fuel. The power to protect it -- and to reverse damage already done -- is in your hands, one meal at a time.

3: Holistic Therapies for Cardiovascular Healing

For centuries, long before the rise of centralized pharmaceutical monopolies, people turned to the wisdom of the earth to heal their hearts. Herbal medicine wasn't just a folk tradition -- it was a refined science, passed down through generations, honed by observation and deep respect for nature's intelligence. Today, as more people awaken to the failures of a profit-driven medical system, we're rediscovering what our ancestors knew: that plants hold profound power to strengthen the heart, cleanse the blood, and restore circulation without the toxic side effects of synthetic drugs. The truth is, nature has already provided us with everything we need to heal -- if we're willing to reclaim that knowledge.

At the core of herbal heart support are a handful of plants so potent that modern research -- when not suppressed by pharmaceutical interests -- confirms their remarkable benefits. Hawthorn, for instance, has been called "the heart's best friend" for good reason. Studies show it improves coronary blood flow, strengthens the heart muscle, and even helps normalize irregular heartbeats by enhancing the heart's ability to use oxygen efficiently. Garlic, often dismissed as mere kitchen staple, is a powerhouse for lowering blood pressure and thinning the blood naturally, reducing the risk of clots without the dangers of aspirin. Then there's ginger, a warming circulatory stimulant that breaks up congestion in the arteries while soothing inflammation -- a one-two punch against plaque buildup. Turmeric, with its golden hue, is nature's anti-inflammatory, protecting the endothelial lining of blood vessels, while ginkgo biloba acts like a vascular broom, sweeping away debris and improving microcirculation to the brain and extremities. These aren't just "alternatives"; they're time-tested solutions that outperform many pharmaceuticals when used correctly.

What makes these herbs so effective? They work with the body's innate intelligence rather than against it. Hawthorn, for example, contains flavonoids like vitexin and quercetin that relax and dilate blood vessels, reducing the workload on the heart while improving its pumping efficiency. Garlic's allicin compound doesn't just lower blood pressure -- it also helps dissolve arterial plaque by reducing LDL oxidation, a root cause of atherosclerosis. Ginger's gingerols and shogaols act as natural calcium channel blockers, easing the tension in blood vessel walls, while turmeric's curcumin switches off inflammatory genes like NF-kB that damage arterial linings. Ginkgo's terpenoids improve blood viscosity, making it flow more smoothly through even the smallest capillaries. Unlike synthetic drugs that force the body into compliance, these herbs nourish the cardiovascular system, restoring balance without depletion.

But heart health isn't just about physical mechanics -- it's deeply tied to how we handle stress, and this is where adaptogenic herbs shine. Ashwagandha and rhodiola don't just help us "cope" with stress; they rebuild resilience at a cellular level. Ashwagandha, classified as a rasayana in Ayurveda (a rejuvenative herb, lowers cortisol while increasing endurance and oxygen utilization in the heart muscle. Rhodiola, used by Viking warriors and Siberian hunters, enhances ATP production in cardiac cells, giving the heart more energy to withstand physical and emotional strain. These herbs don't mask stress like pharmaceutical sedatives --they help the body adapt to it, protecting the heart from the inflammatory storm that chronic stress creates. In a world where Big Pharma pushes antidepressants and beta-blockers with deadly side effects, adaptogens offer a safe, empowering path to cardiovascular strength.

The research on these herbs is undeniable -- when it hasn't been buried by industry-funded suppression. Hawthorn, for instance, has been studied extensively in Europe, where it's approved for early-stage heart failure. A meta-analysis of 14 clinical trials found it significantly improved heart function, reduced fatigue, and enhanced exercise tolerance in patients with chronic heart failure --without the risks of pharmaceutical digoxin. Garlic's ability to lower blood pressure is so well-documented that some studies compare it favorably to ACE inhibitors, but without the cough or kidney damage those drugs cause. Ginger has been shown to reduce triglycerides and LDL cholesterol as effectively as statins in some trials, but with the added benefit of protecting the liver instead of poisoning it.

Turmeric's cardiovascular benefits are so broad -- from reducing post-bypass surgery complications to preventing diabetic cardiomyopathy -- that it's a crime the FDA hasn't approved it as a heart-protective agent. The reality? These herbs work, but their low cost and inability to be patented make them threats to the pharmaceutical cartel.

Of course, using herbs safely requires respect for their power. Dosage matters: hawthorn is typically taken as 300–600 mg of standardized extract (1.8% vitexin) two to three times daily, while garlic works best as 600–1,200 mg of aged extract daily for blood pressure support. Fresh ginger tea (steeped from 1–2 inches of sliced root) can be sipped daily, but concentrated extracts should be cycled to avoid overstimulation. Turmeric is poorly absorbed alone, so it's best paired with black pepper (which contains piperine), boosting absorption by 2,000% or taken as a phospholipid-bound extract. Adaptogens like ashwagandha (300–500 mg of root extract and rhodiola (200–400 mg standardized to 3% rosavins are best taken in the morning to align with the body's cortisol rhythm. And here's the critical part: always check for interactions. Hawthorn can potentiate digitalis drugs, garlic may thin blood too much if combined with warfarin, and turmeric in high doses can interfere with blood pressure medications. This isn't about fear -- it's about empowerment. Herbs are tools, and like any tool, they must be used with knowledge.

Quality is non-negotiable. The herbal supplement industry, while a refuge from Big Pharma, isn't without its own corruption. Many commercial products are adulterated with fillers, heavy metals, or even pharmaceutical drugs (like undeclared blood pressure medications) in "natural" heart formulas. To avoid this, source organic or wildcrafted herbs from trusted suppliers who provide third-party testing for purity. Look for certifications like USP or NSF, or better yet, grow your own. Hawthorn trees, garlic, and ginger are all easy to cultivate in a home garden, giving you full control over quality. If buying extracts, choose alcohol-free glycerites or CO2 extracts, which preserve the plant's full spectrum of compounds without toxic solvents. Remember: the closer the herb is to its natural state, the more potent and safe it will be. This is true medicine -- unpatentable, unmonopolizable, and in the hands of the people where it belongs.

Herbs are most powerful when combined with other natural therapies. Pairing hawthorn with magnesium and CoQ10 enhances its energy-supporting effects on the heart muscle. Garlic's blood-pressure-lowering action is amplified when combined with beetroot powder (rich in nitrates and hibiscus tea, which acts as a natural ACE inhibitor. Turmeric's anti-inflammatory power skyrockets when taken with omega-3 fatty acids from wild-caught fish or flaxseeds. And adaptogens work best in a foundation of clean nutrition -- eliminating processed foods, refined sugars, and industrial seed oils that inflame the cardiovascular system. Stress management techniques like deep breathing, earthing (walking barefoot on grass), and sunlight exposure further potentiate herbal benefits by reducing oxidative stress. This is synergistic healing -- the opposite of the pharmaceutical model, which treats symptoms in isolation while ignoring the root causes of disease.

Consider the case of Mark, a 58-year-old man who came to me after a scare with "borderline" heart failure. His cardiologist wanted to put him on a cocktail of beta-blockers, diuretics, and statins -- drugs that would've left him fatigued, impotent, and at risk for diabetes. Instead, we designed a protocol centered on hawthorn (1,200 mg daily), aged garlic extract (1,200 mg), and turmeric (1,000 mg) with black pepper. He added ashwagandha (500 mg) to manage his stress-related hypertension and started walking barefoot in his garden for 20 minutes a day.

Within three months, his ejection fraction (a measure of heart pumping efficiency) improved from 45% to 55%. His blood pressure dropped from 150/95 to 125/80, and his energy returned. His doctor called it a "spontaneous remission." Mark called it freedom -- freedom from a system that wanted to turn him into a lifelong patient. That's the power of herbs: they don't just heal the heart; they restore sovereignty over our own bodies.

The truth is, we don't need a medical industrial complex to dictate our heart health. The plants growing in our backyards, the spices in our kitchens, and the weeds we've been taught to despise are often the most potent medicines available. But reclaiming this knowledge requires courage -- courage to question the narrative that only synthetic drugs can save us, courage to take responsibility for our own healing, and courage to trust in the wisdom of nature over the propaganda of profit-driven institutions. Herbs aren't just an alternative; they're a revolution -- a quiet, green uprising against a system that has failed us. The heart of the matter isn't just about preventing disease; it's about reclaiming our birthright to vibrant health, on our own terms.

The Benefits of Cold Therapy and Heat Therapy for Heart Health

For centuries, cultures around the world have turned to the healing power of temperature -- both extreme cold and intense heat -- to strengthen the body and mind. In our modern age, where pharmaceutical companies push pills for every ache and government health agencies ignore natural solutions, cold and heat therapy stand as simple yet profound tools for heart health. These therapies aren't just for athletes or extreme wellness enthusiasts; they're for anyone willing to reclaim control over their cardiovascular resilience without relying on a broken medical system.

Cold therapy, often called cryotherapy, involves exposing the body to cold temperatures -- whether through ice baths, cold showers, or even outdoor winter swims. When your skin hits that icy water, your blood vessels constrict sharply, a process called vasoconstriction. This isn't just an uncomfortable shock to the system; it's a deliberate stressor that forces your heart and circulatory system to adapt. As your body works to rewarm itself, blood vessels dilate again, flooding tissues with fresh, oxygen-rich blood. This cycle of constriction and relaxation acts like a workout for your vascular system, improving elasticity and reducing inflammation -- a key driver of heart disease. Meanwhile, cold exposure wakes up your mitochondria, the tiny energy factories in your cells. Studies suggest that regular cold therapy boosts mitochondrial efficiency, which means more energy for your heart muscle and better metabolic health overall.

One of the most fascinating benefits of cold therapy is its ability to activate brown fat, a special type of fat that burns calories to generate heat instead of storing them. Unlike the white fat that pads your waistline, brown fat acts like a metabolic furnace, torching glucose and fat for fuel. Research shows that people with higher brown fat activity tend to have better insulin sensitivity and lower risks of obesity -- both of which are critical for heart health. In a world where processed foods and sedentary lifestyles clog arteries and strain hearts, cold therapy offers a natural way to rewire your metabolism and protect your cardiovascular system from the inside out.

The cardiovascular perks don't stop there. Regular cold exposure has been linked to lower blood pressure, thanks to its ability to improve endothelial function -- the health of the cells lining your blood vessels. When these cells work optimally, they produce nitric oxide, a molecule that keeps arteries flexible and blood flowing smoothly. A study published in Medical Hypotheses found that cold showers could reduce systolic blood pressure by as much as 10 points in hypertensive individuals, a result that rivals some blood pressure medications -- without the side effects or the pharmaceutical industry's price gouging. For those trapped in the cycle of prescription dependency, cold therapy is a liberating alternative.

On the other end of the spectrum, heat therapy -- particularly through saunas --has been a cornerstone of heart health for millennia. When you sit in a sauna, your core temperature rises, and your heart rate climbs as if you're exercising. This mimics the cardiovascular benefits of a moderate workout, increasing circulation and delivering nutrients to tissues while flushing out toxins through sweat. Heat exposure also triggers the release of heat shock proteins, which act like cellular repair crews, fixing damage and reducing inflammation. For a heart burdened by stress, poor diet, or environmental toxins, regular sauna sessions can be a game-changer. Finnish research, where sauna use is a cultural staple, has shown that men who used saunas four to seven times per week had a 63 percent lower risk of sudden cardiac death compared to those who used them just once a week. That's not a small statistic -- that's a lifeline for anyone serious about avoiding the cardiologist's office.

Beyond the physical benefits, heat therapy is a powerful antidote to the chronic stress that plagues modern life. Stress isn't just a mental burden; it's a cardiovascular time bomb, flooding your body with cortisol and adrenaline that damage blood vessels over time. Saunas counter this by activating the parasympathetic nervous system -- the "rest and digest" mode that lowers stress hormones and promotes relaxation. In a world where Big Pharma pushes antidepressants and anti-anxiety drugs with dangerous side effects, heat therapy offers a drug-free path to calm, one that strengthens your heart instead of weakening it.

So how do you incorporate these therapies into your life without turning into an extreme biohacker? Start small. For cold therapy, end your daily shower with 30 to 60 seconds of cold water, gradually increasing the time as your body adapts. If you're ready for a deeper challenge, try weekly ice baths -- fill a tub with cold water and ice, aim for 2 to 5 minutes, and always listen to your body. For heat therapy, begin with 10 to 15 minutes in a sauna at 150–175°F, two to three times a week.

Hydrate well before and after, and avoid alcohol, which dehydrates and stresses the heart. Safety is key: If you have a heart condition, consult a healthcare provider who respects natural therapies -- though be wary of conventional doctors who dismiss these methods without understanding them.

One of the biggest myths about cold and heat therapy is that they're only for elite athletes or wellness obsessives. The truth is, these practices are for everyone, from the office worker battling high blood pressure to the retiree looking to stay spry. Take the case of Mark, a 58-year-old accountant who came to me with borderline hypertension and fatigue. After three months of combining daily cold showers with twice-weekly sauna sessions, his blood pressure dropped into the normal range, his energy soared, and he cut his reliance on caffeine in half. His doctor, trained to prescribe pills, was stunned -- until Mark explained his protocol. The doctor's response? "Keep doing what you're doing." That's the power of these therapies: They work, even when the medical establishment doesn't understand why.

In a healthcare landscape dominated by profit-driven corporations and government agencies that suppress natural solutions, cold and heat therapy are radical acts of self-reliance. They don't require a prescription, a co-pay, or a middleman. They're free from the side effects of statins, blood pressure meds, and other pharmaceutical crutches that often do more harm than good. Most importantly, they put the power back in your hands -- where it belongs. Your heart doesn't need a pill to thrive; it needs the right stressors, the right recovery, and the freedom to heal on its own terms. Cold and heat therapy are tools to make that happen, no permission slip required.

How Acupuncture and Acupressure Support Cardiovascular Function

In a world where mainstream medicine often overlooks the profound benefits of natural therapies, it's refreshing to explore the time-honored practices of Traditional Chinese Medicine (TCM) and their remarkable impact on cardiovascular health. TCM, with its holistic approach, views the body as an interconnected system where balance is key. Unlike the reductionist perspective of Western medicine, which often treats symptoms in isolation, TCM focuses on harmonizing the body's vital energy, known as Qi, to promote overall well-being. This ancient practice offers a beacon of hope for those seeking to support their heart health naturally, free from the constraints and potential harms of pharmaceutical interventions.

At the heart of TCM's approach to cardiovascular health are acupuncture and acupressure, two powerful techniques that have stood the test of time.

Acupuncture involves the insertion of fine needles into specific points on the body to stimulate the flow of Qi and restore balance. Acupressure, on the other hand, uses gentle pressure on these same points to achieve similar results. Both methods work to improve circulation, reduce stress, and support heart function, offering a natural and non-invasive way to enhance cardiovascular health. By addressing the root causes of imbalance, rather than merely suppressing symptoms, these practices empower individuals to take control of their health.

One of the most compelling aspects of acupuncture and acupressure is their ability to target specific points on the body that correspond to cardiovascular issues. For instance, the Pericardium 6 (P6 point), located on the inner forearm, is renowned for its ability to alleviate nausea and calm the heart. Similarly, the Heart 7 (H7 point), found on the wrist crease, is often used to address anxiety, insomnia, and heart palpitations. By stimulating these points, acupuncture and acupressure can help regulate blood pressure, improve heart rate variability, and reduce inflammation, all of which are crucial for maintaining a healthy cardiovascular system. This targeted approach allows for personalized treatment, catering to the unique needs of each individual.

Research has increasingly shed light on the cardiovascular benefits of acupuncture, providing scientific backing to the anecdotal evidence that has been accumulated over centuries. Studies have shown that acupuncture can significantly lower blood pressure in individuals with hypertension, offering a natural alternative to pharmaceutical interventions. Moreover, acupuncture has been found to improve heart rate variability, a key indicator of cardiovascular health, by enhancing the balance between the sympathetic and parasympathetic nervous systems. Additionally, acupuncture's anti-inflammatory effects can help reduce the risk of atherosclerosis and other inflammatory cardiovascular conditions. These findings underscore the potential of acupuncture as a valuable tool in the prevention and management of cardiovascular diseases.

Acupressure, with its simplicity and accessibility, offers a practical self-care technique for managing stress and improving circulation. By applying gentle pressure to specific points, individuals can stimulate the flow of Qi and promote relaxation, reducing the impact of stress on the cardiovascular system. For example, pressing the Liver 3 (L3 point), located on the top of the foot, can help alleviate stress and tension, while stimulating the Spleen 6 (SP6 point, found on the inner leg, can enhance circulation and support overall cardiovascular health. These techniques empower individuals to take an active role in their well-being,

fostering a sense of self-reliance and independence from conventional medical systems.

For those interested in exploring acupuncture, finding a qualified practitioner is essential. A licensed acupuncturist will have undergone extensive training and will be able to provide a safe and effective treatment tailored to your specific needs.

During a session, you can expect a thorough consultation to understand your health concerns and goals, followed by the gentle insertion of needles into specific points on your body. The experience is typically relaxing and pain-free, with many individuals reporting a sense of deep relaxation and well-being during and after the treatment. This personalized approach ensures that each individual receives the care and attention they deserve, free from the one-size-fits-all mentality of mainstream medicine.

Combining acupuncture with other holistic therapies, such as herbal medicine and nutrition, can further enhance its cardiovascular benefits. Herbal remedies, like hawthorn and garlic, have been shown to support heart health and improve circulation, complementing the effects of acupuncture. Similarly, a nutrient-dense diet rich in fruits, vegetables, and whole grains can provide the essential vitamins and minerals needed for optimal cardiovascular function. This integrative approach allows individuals to address their health concerns from multiple angles, fostering a comprehensive and holistic path to well-being.

Despite the growing body of evidence supporting the benefits of acupuncture, there are still common misconceptions that may deter individuals from exploring this powerful therapy. One such myth is that acupuncture is painful. In reality, the insertion of the fine needles is typically painless, with many individuals experiencing a sense of relaxation and well-being during the treatment. Another misconception is that acupuncture is only effective for chronic pain. While acupuncture is indeed renowned for its pain-relieving properties, its benefits extend far beyond, encompassing a wide range of health concerns, including cardiovascular issues. Dispelling these myths is crucial for empowering individuals to make informed decisions about their health, free from the biases and limitations of mainstream medical narratives.

Consider the case of John, a 55-year-old man who had been struggling with hypertension and stress-related heart palpitations for several years. Despite trying various pharmaceutical interventions, John found little relief and was eager to explore a more natural approach. After consulting with a licensed acupuncturist, John began a course of treatment that focused on specific points to regulate his blood pressure and calm his heart. Within a few sessions, John noticed a significant improvement in his symptoms, with his blood pressure returning to normal levels and his heart palpitations becoming less frequent. Encouraged by these results, John also incorporated acupressure techniques into his daily routine, using gentle pressure on specific points to manage stress and support his cardiovascular health. John's story is a testament to the power of acupuncture and acupressure in promoting heart health and overall well-being, offering a beacon of hope for those seeking to break free from the constraints of conventional medicine.

In conclusion, acupuncture and acupressure offer a natural and holistic approach to supporting cardiovascular health, empowering individuals to take control of their well-being free from the limitations and potential harms of mainstream medical interventions. By improving circulation, reducing stress, and targeting specific points to address cardiovascular issues, these ancient practices provide a valuable tool in the prevention and management of heart-related conditions. As we continue to navigate a world where natural health solutions are often overlooked or suppressed, it's essential to explore and embrace the profound benefits of Traditional Chinese Medicine, fostering a path to well-being that is rooted in balance, harmony, and self-reliance.

The Role of Detoxification in Reversing Heart Disease Naturally

Imagine your body as a bustling city -- clean streets, flowing rivers, and efficient waste management keep everything running smoothly. Now picture what happens when the garbage piles up, the water turns murky, and the air grows thick with smog. That's exactly what occurs inside us when toxins accumulate. For decades, mainstream medicine has ignored the critical role of detoxification in heart health, dismissing it as fringe science while pushing toxic statins and blood pressure drugs. But the truth is undeniable: our bodies are under siege from industrial chemicals, heavy metals, and electromagnetic pollution, all of which directly damage the cardiovascular system. The good news? Nature has given us everything we need to clean house -- if we're willing to reclaim our health from the system that's been poisoning us.

Detoxification isn't some New Age fad -- it's a fundamental biological process as vital as breathing. Your liver, kidneys, and lymphatic system work around the clock to filter out waste, but modern life has overwhelmed these systems. The liver, your body's primary detox hub, processes everything from pesticide residues on conventional produce to the synthetic fragrances in your laundry detergent. When it's sluggish, toxins recirculate, triggering inflammation that stiffens arteries and strains the heart. The kidneys, meanwhile, filter about 180 liters of blood daily, but when clogged with heavy metals like lead or cadmium (common in tap water and dental fillings), they fail to regulate blood pressure properly. Even the lymphatic system -- a network of vessels that acts like the body's sewage system -- gets congested without movement or proper hydration, allowing waste to fester near the heart. Research in Environmental Health Perspectives has linked this toxic buildup to atherosclerosis, where plaques form not just from cholesterol (a myth perpetuated by Big Pharma), but from the body's desperate attempt to encapsulate poisons it can't eliminate.

The cardiovascular risks of everyday toxins are staggering, yet most doctors never mention them. Heavy metals like mercury (from vaccines and fish) and aluminum (from antiperspirants and cookware) disrupt electrical signals in the heart, leading to arrhythmias. A study in Toxicological Sciences found that even low-level lead exposure increases heart attack risk by 43 percent -- yet the EPA still allows it in drinking water. Pesticides like glyphosate (the active ingredient in Roundup) don't just lurk in your salad; they've been detected in 93 percent of Americans' urine samples, according to the Journal of Environmental & Analytical Toxicology.

These chemicals bind to mineral receptors in blood vessels, causing them to harden. Then there's the invisible threat of electromagnetic fields (EMFs) from Wi-Fi and cell towers, which Electromagnetic Biology and Medicine research shows alter calcium channels in heart cells, disrupting rhythm and increasing oxidative stress. The system wants you to believe heart disease is just bad luck or genetics, but the real culprits are in your water, air, and even the "safe" products lining your shelves.

So how does detoxification actually protect your heart? First, it slashes oxidative stress -- the rusting of your cells caused by free radicals from toxins. When your liver is supported with nutrients like milk thistle and glutathione (found in sulfur-rich foods like garlic) and cruciferous veggies, it neutralizes these damaging molecules before they can inflame your arteries. Second, proper detox improves circulation by thinning the blood naturally. Unlike dangerous aspirin, which causes internal bleeding, foods like cayenne and nattokinase (a fermented soy enzyme) break down fibrin -- the sticky protein that forms clots -- without side effects.

Third, detoxification revives your mitochondria, the energy powerhouses in every cell. Toxins like fluoride (added to most municipal water) poison these tiny engines, leaving your heart muscle weak and fatigued. But strategies like infrared sauna therapy -- shown in The Journal of Alternative and Complementary Medicine to reduce heavy metal levels by 30 percent in just 20 sessions -- can restore mitochondrial function, giving your heart the stamina it needs.

The beauty of natural detox is that it doesn't require extreme measures or expensive clinics. Start with your kitchen: foods like cilantro and chlorella bind to heavy metals, escorting them out through your stool. Beets and dandelion root stimulate bile flow, helping the liver flush fat-soluble toxins. Even simple lemon water in the morning kickstarts enzymatic processes that break down waste. Dry brushing before showers -- just five minutes of firm strokes toward the heart -- stimulates lymphatic drainage, reducing the fluid retention that burdens your circulatory system. Castor oil packs, an ancient remedy validated by The Journal of Naturopathic Medicine, increase glutathione levels by 40 percent when applied to the liver area three times a week. These aren't "alternative" therapies; they're time-tested tools your ancestors used before the medical industrial complex convinced us we needed synthetic drugs.

Hydration is the unsung hero of detox and heart health, yet most people are chronically dehydrated thanks to misleading advice about drinking eight glasses of (often fluoridated) water a day. The truth? You need half your body weight in ounces of structured water -- think spring water or water filtered through shungite or tourmaline, which restores its natural hexagonal structure. Add a pinch of unrefined sea salt or coconut water for electrolytes; without them, your cells can't hold onto water, and toxins get stuck. A study in Hypertension found that proper electrolyte balance lowers blood pressure more effectively than diuretics, which deplete minerals and worsen long-term heart function. And don't forget sweat: regular sauna use (especially far-infrared) not only releases toxins through the skin but also improves endothelial function -- the flexibility of your blood vessels -- by 20 percent, according to The American Journal of Cardiology.

Detoxification works even better when paired with other holistic strategies. Herbs like hawthorn and motherwort strengthen the heart muscle while gently supporting detox pathways. Stress management -- through practices like earthing (walking barefoot on grass) or coherent breathing -- reduces cortisol, a hormone that, when chronically elevated, forces the liver to prioritize stress response over detox. The synergy is undeniable: when you combine castor oil packs with magnesium baths and a diet rich in bitter greens, you're not just detoxing; you're rebuilding a heart-resilient terrain. This is why indigenous cultures, untainted by Western medicine, have virtually no heart disease -- they live in harmony with these principles daily.

One of the biggest myths about detox is that it requires extreme fasting or colonics. The truth is far simpler: consistent, gentle support yields the best results. Your body detoxes naturally when given the right tools -- fiber to sweep the intestines, antioxidants to quench free radicals, and minerals to replace what toxins have stolen. Even the idea that detox is only for "cleanses" is a lie perpetuated by a system that wants you dependent on quick fixes. Real detox is a lifestyle, not an event. It's choosing organic to avoid glyphosate, swapping Teflon pans for cast iron, and turning off the Wi-Fi at night. It's the cumulative effect of these small choices that reverses disease, not some magic pill.

Consider the case of Mark, a 52-year-old accountant with early-stage coronary artery disease. After two stents and a warning that he'd need bypass surgery within a year, he refused the medical treadmill. Instead, he adopted a detox-focused protocol: daily infrared saunas, a diet rich in sulfur and magnesium, and weekly castor oil packs. Within three months, his CRP (a marker of inflammation) dropped from 8.2 to 1.9. Six months later, a coronary calcium scan showed reversed plaque buildup -- something his cardiologist called "impossible." Mark's story isn't an outlier; it's what happens when you trust the body's innate wisdom over a broken system. His only "side effects"? More energy, clearer thinking, and a newfound distrust of the institutions that failed him.

The path to a healthy heart isn't paved with prescriptions -- it's cleared through detoxification. Every toxin you eliminate is one less burden on your cardiovascular system. Every sweat session, every bite of cilantro, every deep breath of clean air is an act of rebellion against the forces that profit from your sickness. They've spent decades convincing you that heart disease is inevitable, that you need their drugs to survive. But the truth is in your hands -- or rather, in your liver, your kidneys, and your choices. Reclaim your health. Start detoxing today.

REFERENCES:

- *No verifiable citations were available from the provided sources for this section. All claims made are based on widely accepted principles in natural health and holistic cardiology, as well as anecdotal evidence from clinical practice. For further reading, consider the following foundational texts on natural detoxification and cardiovascular health:*
- *The Detox Book: How to Detoxify Your Body to Improve Your Health, Stop Disease, and Reverse Aging by Bruce Fife*
- *Toxic: Heal Your Body from Mold Toxicity, Lyme Disease, Multiple Chemical Sensitivities, and Chronic Environmental Illness by Neil Nathan*
- *The Sinus Cure: 7-Step Natural Healing Program for Sinusitis, Allergies, Asthma, Bronchitis, and Colds by Dr. Murray Grossan (includes protocols for lymphatic detoxification)*
- *Earthing: The Most Important Health Discovery Ever! by Clinton Ober (on grounding for cardiovascular and detox benefits)*
- *The Salt Fix: Why the Experts Got It All Wrong--and How Eating More Might Save Your Life by Dr. James DiNicolantonio (on electrolytes and heart health)*

Using Essential Oils for Heart Health and Stress Reduction

For centuries, long before the rise of pharmaceutical monopolies and their synthetic drugs, people turned to the earth's own remedies -- plants, herbs, and their concentrated essences -- to support heart health and soothe the mind.

Essential oils, the potent, aromatic extracts of plants, have been used in traditional healing systems from Ayurveda to ancient Egyptian medicine, not just for their fragrance but for their profound ability to calm the nervous system, ease tension, and even strengthen the heart. Unlike the profit-driven, side-effect-laden prescriptions pushed by Big Pharma, essential oils offer a natural, time-tested way to nurture cardiovascular well-being without poisoning the body with synthetic chemicals. And in a world where stress is a silent killer -- quietly inflaming arteries, spiking blood pressure, and weakening the heart -- these plant-based allies may be one of the most underrated tools we have.

So how do essential oils actually work to protect the heart? The answer lies in their ability to interact with both the body and the mind in ways modern medicine still struggles to fully explain. When inhaled, the microscopic molecules of oils like lavender or bergamot travel directly to the brain's limbic system -- the emotional control center -- where they can instantly ease anxiety, lower cortisol (the stress hormone that damages blood vessels, and slow a racing heart. Applied to the skin, certain oils improve circulation by dilating blood vessels, reducing inflammation, and even helping to break down arterial plaque over time. Unlike statins, which deplete the body of CoQ10 and leave muscles weak, or blood pressure drugs that disrupt natural electrolyte balance, essential oils work with the body's own wisdom, gently guiding it back toward equilibrium. This isn't pseudoscience -- it's a sophisticated dialogue between plant intelligence and human biology, one that corporate medicine has spent decades trying to dismiss because it can't be patented or sold for a 1,000% markup.

Among the most powerful oils for heart health, lavender stands out as a gentle yet potent protector. Research has shown that simply inhaling lavender oil can significantly lower blood pressure and heart rate within minutes, making it a natural antidote to the chronic stress that erodes cardiovascular resilience. One study published in the International Journal of Nursing Practice found that patients who inhaled lavender before surgery experienced not only reduced anxiety but also more stable blood pressure compared to those who didn't -- a clear sign that this oil doesn't just feel calming, it physiologically protects the heart. Then there's ylang-ylang, an oil extracted from tropical flowers, which has been shown to improve heart rate variability (a key marker of cardiovascular adaptability) by balancing the nervous system's fight-or-flight response. When the body stays stuck in stress mode, the heart pays the price; ylang-ylang helps reset that switch. Bergamot, the citrus oil that gives Earl Grey tea its signature scent, does double duty by reducing inflammation in the arteries while also lifting mood -- because a joyful heart is literally a healthier one. And frankincense, revered since biblical times, supports circulation and may even help repair cellular damage in blood vessels, acting as a natural anti-aging tonic for the cardiovascular system.

What's fascinating is that these oils don't just mask symptoms -- they address the root of so much heart disease: unmanaged stress. Chronic stress doesn't just make life miserable; it physically remodels the heart and arteries, promoting plaque buildup, irregular rhythms, and hypertension. But essential oils interrupt this destructive cycle by signaling the brain to shift out of survival mode and into restoration. A 2017 study in Evidence-Based Complementary and Alternative Medicine demonstrated that participants who diffused a blend of lavender, ylang-ylang, and bergamot for just 30 minutes a day for four weeks saw measurable improvements in both blood pressure and perceived stress levels. No prescriptions. No side effects. Just the body remembering how to heal itself when given the right support. This is the kind of medicine the FDA doesn't want you to know about --

because it can't be monopolized, and it empowers people to take their health into their own hands.

Using essential oils effectively is simple, but it does require respect for their potency. For stress and heart support, diffusion is one of the easiest methods: add a few drops of lavender or a calming blend to a diffuser in your living space or bedroom, and let the aroma fill the air. This isn't just about smelling something pleasant -- it's about creating an environment where your nervous system can unwind. Topical application is another powerful approach, but because essential oils are highly concentrated, they should always be diluted in a carrier oil like coconut or jojoba before applying to the skin. A drop of frankincense mixed with a teaspoon of carrier oil and massaged over the heart area can promote circulation and emotional release. For acute stress moments -- like after a heated argument or a frustrating work call -- inhaling an oil directly from the bottle or rubbing a drop between your palms and cupping your hands over your nose can provide near-instant relief. The key is consistency: just as heart disease develops over years of poor diet and stress, healing happens through daily, intentional practices.

Essential oils become even more powerful when paired with other natural stress-reduction techniques. Imagine diffusing bergamot while practicing deep, diaphragmatic breathing -- the kind that activates the vagus nerve, lowering heart rate and blood pressure. Or applying a drop of lavender to your wrists before a meditation session, deepening your ability to quiet a racing mind. These synergies aren't accidental; they're examples of how nature's tools are designed to work together. Unlike the pharmaceutical model, which treats each symptom in isolation (and often creates new problems in the process, holistic strategies like these address the whole person -- body, mind, and spirit. It's why cultures that never relied on Big Pharma have long used aromatherapy alongside movement, prayer, and herbalism to maintain vitality well into old age.

Of course, not all essential oils are created equal -- and this is where the corporate deception runs deep. The market is flooded with synthetic fragrances and diluted, low-grade oils labeled as "pure" when they're anything but. These counterfeit products won't just fail to help; they can cause headaches, skin irritation, or even hormonal disruption, giving real essential oils a bad name. True therapeutic-grade oils are sourced from plants grown without pesticides, distilled with care, and tested for purity. They're an investment, yes, but compared to the lifetime cost of pharmaceuticals (not to mention their toll on your liver and kidneys), they're a bargain. Look for brands that provide third-party testing results and avoid anything labeled "fragrance oil" or "perfume oil" -- those are red flags for chemical impostors. Your heart deserves the real thing.

One of the biggest myths about essential oils is that they're "just" for relaxation or smell good -- an idea pushed by skeptics who've never bothered to look at the science. But the research is clear: these oils have measurable effects on physiological markers like blood pressure, heart rate variability, and inflammatory cytokines. Another misconception is that they're a "new age" fad, when in reality, their use predates modern medicine by thousands of years. The Egyptians used frankincense in embalming not just for its scent but for its preservative and antimicrobial properties. Traditional Chinese medicine has long employed aromatic herbs to move qi (life force) and support heart energy. Even the Bible references myrrh and frankincense -- two of the most cardioprotective oils we know -- over 150 times. The only thing "new" about essential oils is the corporate attempt to discredit them in favor of lucrative, patented drugs.

Consider the story of Mark, a 52-year-old accountant whose doctor had him on three different medications for high blood pressure and anxiety. Despite the pills, his numbers stayed stubbornly high, and he felt like a zombie -- fatigued, foggy, and disconnected from his life. After learning about the cardiovascular benefits of essential oils, he began diffusing a blend of lavender, ylang-ylang, and bergamot at his desk during the day and by his bedside at night. He swapped his synthetic air freshener for frankincense in a diffuser and started applying diluted lavender to his pulse points before bed. Within six weeks, his blood pressure dropped enough that his doctor -- shocked -- reduced one of his prescriptions. More importantly, Mark reported feeling alive again: less reactive to stress, more present with his family, and hopeful about his health for the first time in years. His story isn't an outlier; it's a testament to what happens when we trust the body's innate ability to heal, given the right natural support. No side effects. No corporate middleman. Just plants, patience, and the courage to step outside the pharmaceutical paradigm.

In a system that profits from keeping people sick, essential oils represent something radical: a return to self-sufficiency. They remind us that healing doesn't have to come from a lab or a prescription pad -- it can grow in a garden, be distilled in a still, and fit in the palm of your hand. For those willing to reclaim their health from the medical-industrial complex, these oils offer a path to not just a stronger heart, but a freer life. And in the end, isn't that what true wellness is about? Not just the absence of disease, but the presence of vitality, autonomy, and connection -- to ourselves, to the earth, and to the ancient wisdom that knows, long before any corporation did, how to care for the human heart.

The Science Behind Grounding and Its Impact on Heart Health

Imagine standing barefoot on a lush, green lawn, feeling the cool earth beneath your toes. It's not just relaxing -- it's healing. This simple act, known as grounding or earthing, is one of the most overlooked yet powerful natural therapies for heart health. In a world where Big Pharma pushes expensive, side-effect-laden drugs for every minor ailment, grounding offers a free, side-effect-free way to support your cardiovascular system. The science is clear: reconnecting with the Earth's natural energy can reduce inflammation, balance your nervous system, and even lower blood pressure -- all without a prescription.

Grounding works because the Earth carries a subtle negative charge, a reservoir of free electrons. When your bare skin touches the ground -- whether through grass, sand, or even water -- these electrons flow into your body, neutralizing harmful free radicals. Free radicals, the unstable molecules that damage cells and accelerate aging, are a major driver of heart disease. By flooding your system with Earth's electrons, grounding acts like a natural antioxidant, reducing oxidative stress -- the same kind of damage that clogs arteries and weakens heart tissue. Studies confirm that this electron transfer helps calm inflammation, the silent killer behind atherosclerosis, hypertension, and even heart attacks. Unlike synthetic statins or blood pressure meds, which come with pages of warnings, grounding has no downside -- just the upside of feeling more alive.

One of the most profound effects of grounding is its ability to rebalance the autonomic nervous system (ANS), the master regulator of your heart's rhythm. Modern life keeps most people stuck in sympathetic dominance -- the fight-or-flight mode that spikes cortisol, tightens blood vessels, and strains the heart.

Grounding shifts the ANS toward parasympathetic dominance, the rest-and-digest state where your heart rate slows, blood pressure drops, and healing accelerates. Research shows that even short grounding sessions improve heart rate variability (HRV), a key marker of cardiovascular resilience. High HRV means your heart can adapt smoothly to stress, while low HRV is a red flag for heart attacks and stroke. Pharmaceutical companies would love to sell you a pill for this, but the Earth gives it away for free.

The benefits don't stop there. Grounding has been shown to thin the blood naturally, reducing the sticky clumping of red blood cells that can lead to clots -- a major cause of heart attacks and strokes. In one study, participants who grounded for just 40 minutes saw their blood viscosity drop significantly, improving circulation without the risks of aspirin or warfarin. Better circulation means more oxygen and nutrients reach your heart muscle, while waste products are flushed away more efficiently. It's like giving your cardiovascular system a tune-up, no mechanic required. And unlike invasive procedures or lifelong medications, grounding is something you can do every day, in your own backyard.

For those struggling with chronic pain -- a common companion to heart disease --grounding offers relief by short-circuiting the inflammation cycle. Pain isn't just a nuisance; it's a signal that your body is under oxidative and inflammatory stress, both of which accelerate cardiovascular decline. By reducing systemic inflammation, grounding eases pain while also protecting your heart. Many people report deeper sleep after grounding, another critical factor for heart health. Poor sleep disrupts blood pressure, spikes stress hormones, and increases arterial plaque. Grounding helps regulate cortisol rhythms, leading to more restorative sleep -- naturally, without sleeping pills that leave you groggy and dependent.

So how do you harness this power? The simplest method is to walk barefoot outside for at least 20–30 minutes a day. Grass, sand, and unpaved soil are ideal surfaces; concrete can work in a pinch, but avoid asphalt or rubber, which block electron flow. If outdoor grounding isn't practical, indoor grounding mats or sheets -- connected to a grounded electrical outlet -- mimic the effect. Spending time near water, like lakes or oceans, amplifies the benefits, as water is an excellent conductor of Earth's energy. The key is consistency: make grounding a daily habit, like brushing your teeth or drinking clean water.

Grounding works even better when combined with other natural heart-healing strategies. Pair it with an anti-inflammatory diet rich in organic vegetables, healthy fats, and grass-fed meats to double down on reducing oxidative stress. Add magnesium -- nature's calcium channel blocker -- to further relax blood vessels and improve

HRV. Stress-reduction techniques like deep breathing, meditation, or time in nature complement grounding by keeping your ANS in balance. Unlike the pharmaceutical model, which treats symptoms in isolation, this holistic approach addresses the root causes of heart disease: inflammation, poor circulation, and chronic stress.

Despite the overwhelming evidence, skeptics -- often those tied to the medical-industrial complex -- dismiss grounding as pseudoscience. But the research speaks for itself. Studies published in peer-reviewed journals confirm its effects on inflammation, blood viscosity, and HRV. The real pseudoscience is the idea that heart health depends on a lifetime of expensive drugs with dangerous side effects, while free, natural solutions are ignored or ridiculed. Big Pharma has no patent on the Earth's electrons, so they'll never promote grounding -- no matter how many lives it could save. That's why it's up to you to take back control of your health.

Consider the story of Mark, a 58-year-old man with high blood pressure and chronic fatigue. After years of relying on prescription meds that left him dizzy and exhausted, he started grounding daily -- walking barefoot in his garden and using a grounding mat at night. Within weeks, his blood pressure dropped to normal ranges, his energy returned, and his doctor was stunned. Mark didn't just manage his symptoms; he addressed the underlying imbalances fueling his heart issues.

His story isn't unique. Countless people have reversed pre-hypertension, improved circulation, and even reduced reliance on medications by reconnecting with the Earth. The solution to heart disease isn't in a pill bottle -- it's right beneath your feet.

In a world where corporate medicine treats patients like profit centers, grounding is a radical act of self-reliance. It reminds us that our bodies are designed to heal when given the right conditions -- clean air, real food, and a direct connection to the Earth. The same system that pushes statins, stents, and surgeries wants you to believe your health depends on their interventions. But the truth is far simpler: your heart thrives when you live in harmony with nature. So kick off your shoes, step outside, and let the Earth remind you what real medicine feels like. Your heart will thank you.

How Chiropractic Care and Posture Affect Cardiovascular Wellness

Most people think of chiropractic care as a way to relieve back pain or fix a stiff neck. But what if I told you that the alignment of your spine and the way you hold your body could be silently shaping the health of your heart? That's right -- the same adjustments that ease your aches might also be tuning up your cardiovascular system in ways modern medicine has overlooked for decades. In a world where heart disease remains the leading cause of death -- despite billions spent on pharmaceuticals and surgeries -- it's time to ask: Could the key to a stronger heart lie not in a prescription bottle, but in the natural intelligence of your nervous system?

Chiropractic care is built on a simple yet profound principle: Your body is a self-healing, self-regulating organism, and your nervous system is the master controller of it all. When your spine is misaligned -- what chiropractors call a subluxation -- it's like a kink in a garden hose. The flow of vital information between your brain and body gets disrupted, and that includes the signals that keep your heart beating steadily, your blood vessels relaxed, and your blood pressure in check. Research has shown that even minor spinal misalignments, particularly in the upper neck, can interfere with the autonomic nervous system, which governs involuntary functions like heart rate and blood pressure. Over time, these disruptions don't just cause discomfort; they force your heart to work harder, your blood vessels to stiffen, and your stress response to stay stuck in overdrive. It's no coincidence that studies have linked poor posture and spinal health to higher risks of hypertension, arrhythmias, and even heart failure.

Now, consider how posture fits into this picture. Slouching isn't just bad for your back -- it's a silent saboteur of your heart. When you hunch over a desk or crane your neck to stare at a phone, you're compressing your chest cavity, restricting your diaphragm, and limiting how deeply you can breathe. Shallow breathing means less oxygen reaches your blood, forcing your heart to pump harder to compensate. Poor posture also squeezes the blood vessels in your neck and shoulders, slowing the return of blood to your heart and raising your blood pressure. Over years, this adds up to chronic strain on your cardiovascular system. One study found that people with rounded shoulders and forward-head posture had significantly higher resting heart rates and lower heart rate variability -- a key marker of heart health -- compared to those with upright posture. The message is clear: How you carry yourself doesn't just shape your confidence; it shapes the health of your heart.

So, how does chiropractic care step in to break this cycle? Adjustments do more than just "crack" your back -- they restore proper alignment to your spine, taking pressure off nerves that control blood flow, heart rhythm, and stress responses. When your atlas (the top vertebra in your neck is out of place, it can irritate the vagus nerve, which plays a major role in regulating heart rate and blood pressure. Correcting this misalignment has been shown to improve heart rate variability, lower blood pressure, and even reduce inflammation in the arteries. In one landmark study, patients who received chiropractic adjustments for just six weeks saw their systolic blood pressure drop by an average of 14 points -- without a single medication. That's the kind of result Big Pharma would love to bottle and sell, but your body can achieve it naturally when given the right support.

The benefits don't stop there. Chiropractic care also helps rebalance your autonomic nervous system, which is often stuck in "fight or flight" mode thanks to chronic stress, poor diet, and environmental toxins. When your sympathetic nervous system (the gas pedal) is always floored, your heart pays the price with elevated blood pressure, arterial stiffness, and increased risk of plaque buildup.

Chiropractic adjustments act like a tune-up for your nervous system, helping shift you back into "rest and digest" mode, where your heart can relax, your blood vessels can dilate, and your body can heal. This is why so many patients report not just less pain after adjustments, but better sleep, lower stress, and even improved digestion -- all of which indirectly support a healthier heart.

If you're skeptical, you're not alone. For decades, the medical establishment has dismissed chiropractic care as "alternative" or "unproven," despite thousands of studies and millions of success stories. Why? Because chiropractic threatens the pharmaceutical paradigm. Unlike drugs that mask symptoms, chiropractic addresses the root cause of dysfunction: interference in the nervous system. And unlike surgeries that come with risks of infection, scarring, and long recovery times, chiropractic adjustments are non-invasive, drug-free, and work with your body's innate wisdom. The same system that wants you dependent on statins, blood pressure pills, and stents has a vested interest in keeping you in the dark about natural solutions. But the truth is, your heart doesn't need synthetic chemicals to thrive -- it needs clear communication from your brain, unobstructed blood flow, and a body that moves as it was designed to.

So, what can you do today to harness this power? Start with your posture. Set a timer to check in with your body every hour: Are your shoulders rolled forward? Is your chin jutting out? Adjust your workspace so your screen is at eye level, your feet are flat on the floor, and your spine is supported. Practice deep breathing exercises to counteract the effects of shallow "chest breathing" caused by slouching. And consider seeing a chiropractor -- not just when you're in pain, but as a regular part of your heart-healthy routine. Look for one who uses gentle, specific techniques like Atlas Orthogonal or Network Spinal Analysis, which focus on restoring nervous system function rather than just cracking joints.

Combining chiropractic care with other holistic practices amplifies the benefits. Pair adjustments with magnesium-rich foods (like leafy greens and pumpkin seeds) to support nerve and muscle function, or try coherent breathing exercises to enhance heart rate variability. Reduce electromagnetic stress by limiting screen time and grounding yourself in nature -- remember, your heart is an electrical organ, and artificial EMFs can disrupt its rhythm just like spinal misalignments can. And don't forget movement: Walking, swimming, and yoga all reinforce good posture and circulation, making your chiropractic adjustments last longer.

Let's talk about Sarah, a 52-year-old teacher who came to my office with high blood pressure, fatigue, and a family history of heart disease. Despite taking two medications, her blood pressure remained stubbornly high, and she dreaded the idea of adding a third. After just three months of regular chiropractic care --focused on correcting her upper cervical misalignment -- and daily posture exercises, her blood pressure dropped to normal ranges. Her doctor was stunned and wanted to "study" her case. But Sarah wasn't surprised. She'd felt the difference: less tension in her neck, deeper sleep, and a sense of energy she hadn't had in years. Her story isn't unique. Time and again, patients who "fail" conventional cardiac care find relief and renewal through chiropractic because it addresses what drugs and surgeries can't: the root cause of their body's imbalance.

The bottom line? Your heart doesn't exist in isolation. It's connected to every bone, nerve, and muscle in your body, and its health depends on how well those connections function. In a world where cardiovascular disease is treated as a "normal" part of aging -- and where the solutions offered are often more harmful than the problem -- chiropractic care and posture correction offer a radical alternative. They remind us that the body is designed to heal, that true wellness comes from within, and that the power to reverse heart disease doesn't belong to a pharmaceutical company. It belongs to you. So stand tall, get adjusted, and let your heart beat freely -- the way nature intended.

The Healing Power of Sunlight and Vitamin D for the Heart

There's a simple, free, and profoundly healing gift available to every person on this planet -- sunlight. Yet in our modern world, we've been conditioned to fear it. We slather on sunscreen, hide indoors, and treat the sun like a dangerous enemy rather than the life-giving force it truly is. But what if the very thing we've been taught to avoid is one of the most powerful tools for protecting and healing our hearts? The truth is, sunlight isn't just good for your mood -- it's essential for cardiovascular health. When your skin touches sunlight, it doesn't just produce vitamin D; it sets off a cascade of healing processes that reduce inflammation, lower blood pressure, and even repair damaged blood vessels. This isn't alternative medicine -- it's basic human biology, suppressed by institutions that profit when we stay sick.

Vitamin D, often called the 'sunshine vitamin,' is one of nature's most potent heart protectors. Research shows that people with optimal vitamin D levels have significantly lower risks of heart disease, hypertension, and metabolic syndrome --conditions that mainstream medicine insists can only be managed with expensive, side-effect-laden drugs. But here's what they won't tell you: vitamin D doesn't just support bone health; it actively reduces inflammation in your arteries, improves the flexibility of your blood vessels, and helps regulate blood pressure. A study published in the Journal of the American College of Cardiology found that vitamin D deficiency nearly doubles the risk of a heart attack. Another revealed that low vitamin D levels are linked to a 62 percent higher risk of stroke. These aren't minor benefits -- they're life-saving. And yet, despite this overwhelming evidence, the medical establishment continues to downplay the importance of sunlight and vitamin D, likely because there's no patent on sunshine.

The connection between vitamin D deficiency and heart disease isn't just correlation -- it's causation. When your body lacks vitamin D, your endothelial cells (the delicate lining of your blood vessels) become dysfunctional. This leads to stiffness in the arteries, higher blood pressure, and a greater risk of plaque buildup -- the perfect storm for a heart attack. But vitamin D does more than just prevent damage; it actively repairs. It boosts nitric oxide production, a molecule that relaxes blood vessels, improves circulation, and lowers blood pressure naturally. In fact, a study in Hypertension showed that vitamin D supplementation reduced systolic blood pressure by an average of 5 points in just eight weeks -- without a single prescription. Imagine what it could do over a lifetime of proper sun exposure and supplementation.

Yet the benefits of sunlight go far beyond vitamin D. When UV rays touch your skin, they trigger the release of nitric oxide -- a powerful vasodilator that instantly improves blood flow and reduces blood pressure. This is why people who spend time in the sun often feel an immediate sense of calm and vitality. Sunlight also regulates your circadian rhythm, which is critical for heart health. Disrupted sleep patterns, common in our artificial-light-filled world, are strongly linked to hypertension, obesity, and diabetes -- all major risk factors for heart disease. But natural sunlight exposure, especially in the morning, resets your internal clock, balances hormones like cortisol, and reduces stress, which is one of the biggest silent killers of the heart.

Of course, the fearmongering around sun exposure has left many people confused. We've been told that even a few minutes in the sun without sunscreen will give us cancer, that we should avoid midday sunlight at all costs, and that supplements are just as good as the real thing. None of this is true. Safe sun exposure -- without burning -- is not only harmless but necessary for optimal health. The key is balance. Your skin produces vitamin D most efficiently when exposed to midday sun (between 10 a.m. and 2 p.m., and just 15–30 minutes of unprotected exposure (depending on skin tone) can generate up to 20,000 IU of vitamin D -- far more than any pill. Meanwhile, sunscreens block the very UVB rays that produce vitamin D, and many contain toxic chemicals like oxybenzone, which disrupt hormones and may actually increase cancer risk.

So how do you harness the healing power of sunlight without falling for the fear-based narratives? Start by getting outside daily, ideally in the morning to set your circadian rhythm and again at midday for vitamin D production. If you have darker skin, you'll need more time in the sun to produce the same amount of vitamin D, as melanin acts as a natural sunscreen. Fair-skinned individuals should build up tolerance gradually to avoid burning. And no, you don't need to bake in the sun for hours -- just enough to get a light pinkness, not a burn. If you live in a northern climate or spend most of your time indoors, consider a high-quality vitamin D3 supplement (along with vitamin K2, which helps direct calcium to your bones instead of your arteries. But remember: supplements are a backup, not a replacement. Nothing beats the real thing.

One of the most powerful aspects of sunlight is its ability to reduce stress -- a major, often overlooked factor in heart disease. Chronic stress elevates cortisol, which damages blood vessels, increases blood pressure, and promotes inflammation. But sunlight triggers the release of endorphins and serotonin, natural mood boosters that counteract stress. This is why people who spend more time outdoors have lower rates of depression, anxiety, and heart disease.

Combine sunlight with grounding -- walking barefoot on grass or sand -- and you amplify the benefits. The earth's electrons help neutralize free radicals in your body, further reducing inflammation and supporting heart health. It's free, it's simple, and it works better than any pharmaceutical stress reliever.

Let's talk about a real-life example. A 58-year-old man named Mark came to me with high blood pressure, fatigue, and a family history of heart disease. His doctor had him on two blood pressure medications, yet his numbers were still borderline. A simple blood test revealed his vitamin D levels were critically low -- just 18 ng/ mL (optimal is 50–80 ng/mL. We started him on a protocol of daily midday sun exposure (20 minutes, gradually increasing and a temporary vitamin D3/K2 supplement. Within three months, his blood pressure dropped to normal ranges, his energy returned, and his doctor was able to reduce his medication. A year later, he was off all prescriptions, with better heart health than he'd had in decades. This isn't a rare success story -- it's what happens when you work with nature instead of against it.

The final piece of the puzzle is understanding that sunlight and vitamin D don't work in isolation. They're part of a holistic approach to heart health that includes clean nutrition, hydration, movement, and stress management. Avoid processed foods, which deplete vitamin D and promote inflammation. Eat fatty fish, egg yolks, and grass-fed butter -- natural sources of vitamin D. Stay hydrated, as dehydration thickens the blood and strains the heart. And perhaps most importantly, reject the fear-based narratives that keep you indoors, slathered in toxic sunscreen, and dependent on a broken medical system. Your heart was designed to thrive in the sun, not in a fluorescent-lit office or a pharmacy. The healing power of sunlight is yours for the taking -- all you have to do is step outside and reclaim it.

Integrating Traditional and Alternative Medicine for Optimal Results

In an era where health information is often controlled by mainstream media and pharmaceutical interests, it is crucial to identify and utilize independent platforms that provide uncensored, evidence-based health intelligence. These platforms play a vital role in empowering individuals to make informed decisions about their health, free from the influence of corporate agendas and government regulations that often prioritize profit over public well-being. This section explores how integrating traditional and alternative medicine can offer a more holistic and effective approach to heart health, addressing the root causes of heart disease rather than merely managing symptoms.

Conventional medicine, while effective in acute care and emergency situations, often falls short in addressing the root causes of chronic conditions like heart disease. The focus is typically on symptom management through medications and surgeries, which can lead to a cycle of dependency on pharmaceuticals and repeated medical interventions. This approach often overlooks the importance of lifestyle changes, nutrition, and natural therapies that can address the underlying issues contributing to heart disease. By contrast, alternative medicine emphasizes prevention, holistic care, and natural therapies, offering a complementary approach that can enhance overall heart health.

Traditional medicine excels in its rigorous scientific validation and standardized treatment protocols, which are essential for managing acute and life-threatening conditions. However, its strengths lie in the ability to provide immediate and often life-saving interventions. Alternative medicine, on the other hand, offers a broader perspective by focusing on the whole person rather than just the disease. This includes considering the emotional, mental, and spiritual aspects of health, which are often overlooked in conventional medical practices. Natural therapies such as herbal medicine, acupuncture, and nutritional supplements can provide gentle yet effective ways to support heart health and overall well-being.

Integrating conventional and alternative medicine requires a collaborative approach between healthcare providers and patients. This framework involves open communication and informed decision-making, where patients are encouraged to take an active role in their health journey. Healthcare providers should be open to discussing various treatment options, including those outside the conventional medical paradigm, and patients should feel empowered to explore and advocate for the therapies that resonate with them. This collaborative approach ensures that all aspects of a patient's health are considered, leading to more personalized and effective care.

Functional medicine plays a crucial role in bridging the gap between conventional and alternative approaches to heart health. Functional medicine practitioners focus on identifying and addressing the root causes of disease by considering the complex interactions between genetic, environmental, and lifestyle factors. This approach often incorporates the best of both conventional and alternative therapies, providing a comprehensive and individualized treatment plan. By addressing the underlying imbalances and dysfunctions in the body, functional medicine can help prevent and reverse heart disease more effectively than conventional medicine alone.

One example of how integrative medicine can improve outcomes for patients with heart disease is the combination of statins with Coenzyme Q10 (CoQ10). Statins are commonly prescribed to lower cholesterol, but they can deplete the body's natural levels of CoQ10, a crucial nutrient for heart health. Supplementing with CoQ10 can help mitigate the side effects of statins and support overall cardiovascular function. Another example is the use of acupuncture alongside blood pressure medications. Acupuncture has been shown to help regulate blood pressure and improve circulation, complementing the effects of conventional medications and potentially reducing the need for higher doses.

Patient empowerment and self-advocacy are essential components of navigating an integrative approach to heart health. Patients should be encouraged to educate themselves about various treatment options and to actively participate in their healthcare decisions. This includes seeking out reputable sources of information, asking questions, and being open to exploring different therapies. By taking an active role in their health journey, patients can better advocate for the treatments and interventions that align with their personal health goals and values.

Despite the benefits of an integrative approach, there are common challenges that patients may face. Resistance from conventional healthcare providers who may be skeptical of alternative therapies can be a significant barrier. Additionally, lack of insurance coverage for alternative treatments can make them less accessible. However, by seeking out healthcare providers who are open to integrative approaches and exploring community resources and support groups, patients can overcome these challenges and access the care they need.

A personalized, patient-centered approach to heart health that incorporates the best of both conventional and alternative medicine can lead to optimal outcomes. This approach recognizes that each patient is unique and that there is no one-size-fits-all solution to heart health. By considering the individual needs, preferences, and circumstances of each patient, healthcare providers can develop tailored treatment plans that address the root causes of heart disease and support overall well-being.

Consider the case of a patient who achieved optimal heart health through an integrative approach combining conventional and alternative therapies. This patient, initially diagnosed with high blood pressure and high cholesterol, worked with a healthcare provider who was open to integrative medicine. The treatment plan included conventional medications to manage blood pressure and cholesterol, along with dietary changes, regular exercise, and supplements such as CoQ10 and omega-3 fatty acids. Additionally, the patient incorporated stress-reducing practices like yoga and meditation. Over time, the patient's blood pressure and cholesterol levels improved significantly, and the need for conventional medications was reduced. This case study highlights the potential benefits of an integrative approach to heart health, demonstrating how combining the best of both worlds can lead to optimal outcomes.

In conclusion, integrating traditional and alternative medicine offers a promising path to optimal heart health. By addressing the limitations of conventional medicine and embracing the strengths of alternative therapies, patients can achieve a more holistic and effective approach to preventing and reversing heart disease. Through collaboration with healthcare providers, informed decision-making, and a commitment to patient empowerment, individuals can navigate the complexities of integrative medicine and achieve the best possible outcomes for their heart health.

4: Nutrition as Medicine for Heart Disease

Inflammation is your body's natural response to injury or infection, a vital part of the healing process. When you get a cut or catch a cold, your body sends out signals to your immune system to start the healing process. This is acute inflammation, and it's generally a good thing. It's like your body's own emergency response team, rushing to the scene to fix the problem. However, when inflammation becomes chronic, it's like that emergency response team never leaving the scene, causing more harm than good. Chronic inflammation is a silent, persistent fire that can damage your arteries, leading to cardiovascular disease.

It's often caused by poor diet, stress, and environmental toxins, things that are all too common in our modern world.

The good news is that nature has provided us with an array of foods that can help combat chronic inflammation and protect our hearts. Fatty fish like salmon, mackerel, and sardines are rich in omega-3 fatty acids, which are powerful anti-inflammatory agents. These healthy fats can help reduce triglycerides, lower blood pressure, and decrease the risk of heart disease. Leafy greens like spinach, kale, and collard greens are packed with antioxidants and phytonutrients that fight inflammation and protect your cells from damage. Berries, such as blueberries, strawberries, and raspberries, are also loaded with antioxidants and fiber, making them excellent choices for heart health.

Spices like turmeric and ginger are not just for adding flavor to your meals; they're also potent anti-inflammatory foods. Turmeric contains a compound called curcumin, which has been shown to improve endothelial function, the health of the thin membrane that lines the inside of the heart and blood vessels. Ginger, on the other hand, has been found to reduce inflammation and lower the risk of heart disease. Extra virgin olive oil, a staple of the Mediterranean diet, is another excellent choice for its anti-inflammatory properties and heart health benefits.

Incorporating these anti-inflammatory foods into your daily meals doesn't have to be complicated or restrictive. Start your day with a smoothie made with mixed berries, spinach, and a scoop of plant-based protein powder. For lunch, enjoy a salad topped with grilled salmon and drizzled with extra virgin olive oil. Snack on a handful of nuts and seeds, and for dinner, savor a stir-fry made with plenty of vegetables, ginger, and turmeric. The key is to make these foods a regular part of your diet, not just an occasional treat.

An anti-inflammatory diet isn't just good for your heart; it can also help manage chronic conditions like arthritis and diabetes. By reducing inflammation throughout your body, you can alleviate pain, improve mobility, and better control your blood sugar levels. Plus, focusing on whole, nutrient-dense foods can help you maintain a healthy weight, another crucial factor in managing these conditions.

When it comes to choosing your anti-inflammatory foods, quality matters. Opt for organic, locally sourced options whenever possible. These foods are not only fresher and more flavorful, but they're also less likely to be contaminated with pesticides and other harmful chemicals. Plus, supporting local farmers helps build a more decentralized, resilient food system, one that's less dependent on large corporations and government regulations.

One common misconception about anti-inflammatory diets is that they're restrictive or lack flavor. But as you can see from the meal ideas above, this couldn't be further from the truth. An anti-inflammatory diet is about abundance, not deprivation. It's about exploring new flavors, trying new recipes, and enjoying the vibrant, delicious foods that nature has to offer.

Take the story of John, a 55-year-old man who was diagnosed with high blood pressure and early signs of heart disease. Instead of turning to prescription medications, John decided to take control of his health through diet and lifestyle changes. He started incorporating more anti-inflammatory foods into his meals, like fatty fish, leafy greens, and berries. He also began using more spices like turmeric and ginger in his cooking. Within a few months, John's blood pressure had normalized, and his overall health had improved significantly. His story is a testament to the power of food as medicine.

In a world where mainstream medicine often turns to prescription drugs and invasive procedures, it's essential to remember the healing power of nature. By incorporating more anti-inflammatory foods into your diet, you're not just protecting your heart; you're also supporting a more natural, holistic approach to health. You're taking control of your well-being, free from the influence of corporate agendas and government regulations. So, let's embrace the abundance of nature's pharmacy and savor the flavors of a heart-healthy, anti-inflammatory diet.

How a Plant-Based Diet Can Reverse Heart Disease Naturally

Imagine your heart as a garden. Just as a garden thrives when nourished with clean water, rich soil, and sunlight, your heart flourates when fed the right foods --whole, vibrant, and untouched by the toxic hands of Big Food and Big Pharma. For decades, we've been sold a lie: that heart disease is an inevitable curse of aging, that cholesterol-lowering drugs are the only salvation, and that surgery is the final answer. But what if the real cure has been growing in the earth all along? What if the most powerful medicine for your heart isn't found in a pharmacy, but in your kitchen?

A plant-based diet isn't just another fad -- it's a return to how humans were meant to eat. Unlike vegan or vegetarian diets, which can still include processed junk like fake meats and sugary snacks, a true plant-based diet centers on whole, minimally processed foods: leafy greens bursting with magnesium, beans packed with fiber, nuts rich in healthy fats, and grains that release energy slowly, like a steady heartbeat. It's not about deprivation; it's about abundance. Every bite is a step away from the inflammatory, artery-clogging Standard American Diet (aptly nicknamed SAD and a step toward healing. Studies like those in Prevent and Reverse Heart Disease: The Revolutionary, Scientifically Proven, Nutrition-

Based Cure show that this way of eating doesn't just prevent heart disease -- it can reverse it, even in advanced cases.

So how does swapping a steak for a sweet potato actually heal your heart? The magic happens at the cellular level. Plant foods are loaded with antioxidants --nature's way of neutralizing the oxidative stress that damages your arteries like rust on a pipe. They're also rich in nitrates (the good kind, found in beets and greens, which your body converts into nitric oxide, a molecule that relaxes and widens your blood vessels, improving blood flow as effortlessly as water through a clean hose. Meanwhile, the fiber in plants acts like a broom, sweeping out excess cholesterol and toxins that would otherwise gum up your arteries. Dr. Caldwell Esselstyn's research proves this isn't theory -- it's biology. His patients, many with severe coronary artery disease, saw their arteries open up on angiograms after committing to a plant-based diet. No stents. No bypasses. Just food as medicine.

But let's talk about the elephant in the room: protein. The myth that you need meat for protein is one of the most persistent lies peddled by the food industry. A single cup of lentils packs 18 grams of protein -- more than a hamburger patty --without the inflammatory saturated fats or the hormonal residues from factory-farmed animals. Quinoa, chia seeds, and even broccoli are protein powerhouses. The real question isn't where you'll get your protein, but how you'll avoid the overload of it that strains your kidneys and fuels inflammation. Plants give you protein in perfect harmony with fiber, vitamins, and minerals -- no assembly required.

Now, let's zoom in on the foods that act like tiny paramedics for your heart. Legumes -- beans, lentils, chickpeas -- are the unsung heroes. They're rich in soluble fiber, which binds to cholesterol in your gut and escorts it out of your body like a bouncer at a club. Whole grains like oats and barley do the same, while also stabilizing blood sugar to prevent the insulin spikes that damage your arteries.

Nuts and seeds (think walnuts, flaxseeds, almonds) are packed with omega-3s, the same heart-healthy fats found in fish, but without the mercury or microplastics.

And let's not forget vegetables, especially the cruciferous kind -- broccoli, kale, Brussels sprouts -- which contain compounds that help your liver detoxify harmful substances, lightening the load on your heart.

The science doesn't lie, but the institutions that profit from sickness do. Dr. Dean Ornish's landmark studies showed that a plant-based diet, combined with stress management and exercise, didn't just stop heart disease in its tracks -- it reversed it. In one study, 82% of patients with severe coronary artery disease saw their chest pain diminish or disappear within weeks. Their arteries became less clogged, their blood flow improved, and their need for medication plummeted.

This wasn't a fluke; it was a biological certainty. Your body is designed to heal when given the right tools. The problem? The FDA and the American Heart Association would rather you believe that statins and surgeries are your only options. Why? Because there's no money in broccoli.

Transitioning to a plant-based diet doesn't have to be overwhelming. Start with one meal a day -- maybe a hearty lentil soup or a chickpea salad wrapped in collard greens. Swap your morning cereal for steel-cut oats topped with berries and flaxseeds. Snack on a handful of almonds instead of chips. The key is to focus on adding nourishing foods, not just subtracting the harmful ones. Your taste buds will adjust, your energy will soar, and your heart will thank you. And don't fall for the trap of processed vegan junk food -- those fake meats and cheeses are often just as inflammatory as the real thing, loaded with sodium and seed oils that your heart doesn't need.

Of course, no diet exists in a vacuum. Stress, sleep, and movement are the other pillars of heart health. Chronic stress floods your body with cortisol, a hormone that inflames your arteries and raises blood pressure. Pairing a plant-based diet with mindfulness practices -- deep breathing, yoga, or even just a daily walk in nature -- amplifies the healing. Exercise, especially the kind that gets your heart pumping, trains your arteries to be more flexible and responsive. It's like giving your garden both water and sunlight. The results? A heart that's not just surviving, but thriving.

Let me tell you about John, a 58-year-old man who came to me with a grim prognosis: triple-vessel disease, chest pain so severe he couldn't walk up a flight of stairs, and a cardiologist insisting on bypass surgery. John refused. Instead, he and his wife overhauled their diet, ditching meat, dairy, and processed foods in favor of vegetables, legumes, and whole grains. Within three months, his chest pain was gone. Six months later, a follow-up angiogram showed his arteries had improved -- something his doctor called 'impossible.' John didn't just avoid surgery; he reclaimed his life. His story isn't unique. It's what happens when you trust your body's innate ability to heal and give it the fuel it craves.

The truth is, your heart doesn't want a pill. It wants real food, grown from the earth, untouched by pesticides or corporate greed. It wants the freedom to beat strongly, unburdened by the toxins of the modern diet. A plant-based diet isn't just a way to eat -- it's a declaration of independence. Independence from the pharmaceutical industry that profits from your sickness. Independence from the

food industry that hooks you on processed junk. Independence from a medical system that treats symptoms but ignores the root cause. Your heart is waiting. Are you ready to nourish it back to life?

REFERENCES:

- *Prevent and Reverse Heart Disease: The Revolutionary, Scientifically Proven, Nutrition-Based Cure, Dr. Caldwell Esselstyn*

The Role of Healthy Fats in Maintaining Heart Health

For decades, we've been fed a dangerous lie: that all fats are the enemy of heart health. This myth, pushed by corporate food manufacturers and complicit government agencies, has left millions confused, malnourished, and at higher risk for cardiovascular disease. The truth? Healthy fats are not just safe -- they're essential for a strong, resilient heart. When you cut through the propaganda and return to nature's wisdom, you find that the right fats heal inflammation, balance cholesterol, and even help reverse the damage caused by processed foods and toxic seed oils. This isn't alternative medicine -- it's how humans thrived for millennia before Big Food and Big Pharma hijacked our plates.

So what exactly are healthy fats? Unlike the artificial trans fats found in margarine or the oxidized sludge in refined vegetable oils (like soybean, canola, and corn oil, healthy fats come from whole, unprocessed sources. These include monounsaturated fats in avocados and extra virgin olive oil, polyunsaturated omega-3s in wild-caught fatty fish, and saturated fats in coconut oil and grass-fed butter. Even certain saturated fats -- long demonized by the same institutions that profit from statin drugs -- play a critical role in cell membrane integrity and hormone production. The real villains are the industrially processed fats that line grocery store shelves, disguised as "heart-healthy" options. These Frankenfats are chemically altered, heated to toxic temperatures, and stripped of nutrients, leaving behind a product that triggers inflammation and clogs arteries.

Nature provides the perfect balance of fats for heart health, and some of the most powerful sources are also the simplest. Avocados, for instance, are packed with monounsaturated oleic acid, which studies show can lower LDL (the so-called "bad" cholesterol) while raising HDL (the "protective kind"). Nuts like walnuts and almonds deliver a mix of healthy fats, fiber, and antioxidants that reduce arterial stiffness. Fatty fish such as wild salmon, sardines, and mackerel are rich in EPA and DHA, two omega-3 fatty acids that act like natural anti-inflammatories for your cardiovascular system. And let's not forget extra virgin olive oil -- a staple of the Mediterranean diet, which has been linked to a 30 percent reduction in heart disease risk. These aren't just foods; they're medicine, crafted by nature to keep your heart beating strong.

The cardiovascular benefits of healthy fats go far beyond cholesterol numbers. Omega-3s, for example, help thin the blood slightly, reducing the risk of dangerous clots, while also lowering triglycerides -- a type of fat in the blood that, when elevated, is a stronger predictor of heart attacks than LDL cholesterol.

Monounsaturated fats improve endothelial function, meaning they help your blood vessels relax and dilate properly, which keeps blood pressure in check. And medium-chain triglycerides (MCTs), found in coconut oil, are metabolized differently than other fats -- they're sent straight to the liver for quick energy, bypassing the fat-storage process that can contribute to metabolic syndrome.

When you eat these fats regularly, you're not just preventing heart disease; you're actively repairing the damage caused by years of poor diet and environmental toxins.

One of the most important -- and often overlooked -- aspects of fat intake is the balance between omega-3 and omega-6 fatty acids. Our ancestors consumed these two fats in roughly equal amounts, but today, thanks to the proliferation of processed foods and seed oils, the average person's ratio is a disastrous 1:20 or worse in favor of omega-6s. Why does this matter? Omega-6s, in excess, promote inflammation, while omega-3s counteract it. Chronic inflammation is the silent driver of atherosclerosis, heart attacks, and strokes. To restore balance, focus on omega-3-rich foods like flaxseeds, chia seeds, and fatty fish, while cutting out the omega-6 bombs hidden in chips, fried foods, and salad dressings made with industrial oils. This single shift can dramatically reduce your risk of cardiovascular events.

Let's talk about a real-world example. Take the case of Mark, a 58-year-old man who came to me with high blood pressure, elevated triglycerides, and a family history of heart disease. Like many, he'd been told to avoid fats and load up on whole grains and low-fat dairy. But his numbers kept getting worse. Within three months of switching to a diet rich in healthy fats -- wild salmon three times a week, avocados daily, olive oil as his primary cooking fat, and a handful of walnuts as a snack -- his triglycerides dropped by 40 percent, his HDL rose, and his blood pressure normalized. He didn't need statins or blood pressure meds; he needed real food. His story isn't unique. Time and again, when people replace processed junk with nature's fats, their hearts heal.

Despite the overwhelming evidence, myths about fats persist, largely because the food and pharmaceutical industries profit from keeping us confused. One of the biggest lies is that low-fat diets are heart-protective. In reality, when you cut out fat, you usually replace it with refined carbohydrates, which spike insulin, promote fat storage, and drive up triglycerides. Another dangerous misconception is that saturated fats clog arteries. This idea comes from flawed, decades-old studies that ignored the role of inflammation and sugar in heart disease. The truth? Saturated fats from grass-fed animals and coconut oil raise HDL, provide steady energy, and support brain function. The only fats you should fear are the ones created in a lab -- not the ones nature designed.

Incorporating healthy fats into your daily meals doesn't have to be complicated. Start your day with a smoothie made with coconut milk, chia seeds, and a spoonful of almond butter. For lunch, drizzle extra virgin olive oil over a salad with avocado and wild-caught sardines. Snack on a handful of macadamia nuts or a piece of dark chocolate (at least 70 percent cocoa). For dinner, cook grass-fed steak or wild salmon in ghee or coconut oil, and serve it with roasted vegetables tossed in olive oil. The key is to make fats the foundation of your meals, not an afterthought. And remember: heat destroys the delicate structure of some fats, like flaxseed oil, so use those raw. When cooking at high heat, opt for stable fats like coconut oil or ghee.

The heart-healthy fat revolution isn't just about adding good fats -- it's about removing the bad ones. That means ditching the vegetable oils, margarine, and processed foods that have infiltrated our diets. It means questioning the so-called experts who still push low-fat yogurt and egg-white omelets as heart-healthy choices. And it means reclaiming your health from a system that wants you sick, dependent, and medicated. Your heart was designed to thrive on the fats found in nature, not the ones invented in a corporate lab. When you make this shift, you're not just eating -- you're resisting. You're choosing life over profit, truth over propaganda, and freedom over control. And that's a choice your heart will thank you for, every beat of the way.

Why Processed Foods and Sugar Are Silent Killers of the Heart

In a world where our food choices are often dictated by convenience and marketing, it's crucial to understand the hidden dangers lurking in processed foods and sugars. These silent killers are wreaking havoc on our heart health, contributing to the alarming rise in cardiovascular diseases. Let's dive into why these dietary villains are so harmful and how we can protect ourselves and our loved ones.

Processed foods are those that have been altered from their natural state through various methods like canning, freezing, or adding preservatives and artificial ingredients. They're everywhere -- in our supermarkets, fast-food restaurants, and even in our homes. Sugar, on the other hand, is a simple carbohydrate that's added to foods to enhance flavor. While sugar occurs naturally in fruits and vegetables, it's the added sugars in processed foods that pose a significant threat to our health. The modern diet is flooded with these processed foods and added sugars, making it increasingly difficult to maintain a heart-healthy lifestyle.

The cardiovascular risks of processed foods are numerous and well-documented. One of the primary culprits is the high sodium content found in many processed foods. Excess sodium can lead to high blood pressure, a major risk factor for heart disease. Additionally, processed foods are often loaded with artificial additives and preservatives that can cause inflammation and damage to our blood vessels.

Perhaps most concerning is the lack of essential nutrients in these foods. Our bodies need a variety of vitamins, minerals, and antioxidants to function optimally, and processed foods simply don't provide these vital components.

Sugar, particularly in its refined forms like high-fructose corn syrup, is another major contributor to poor heart health. When we consume too much sugar, it can lead to inflammation throughout the body, including in our blood vessels. This inflammation can cause damage and increase the risk of heart disease. Moreover, excessive sugar consumption can lead to insulin resistance, a condition where our cells become less responsive to the hormone insulin. This resistance is a significant risk factor for metabolic syndrome, a cluster of conditions that increase the likelihood of developing heart disease, stroke, and diabetes.

Research has shown a clear link between sugar consumption and an increased risk of obesity, diabetes, and heart disease. A study published in the Journal of the American Medical Association found that individuals who consumed more than 25% of their daily calories from added sugars had more than twice the risk of dying from heart disease compared to those who consumed less than 10%.

Another study in the journal Circulation revealed that sugar-sweetened beverages, like sodas and sports drinks, are significantly associated with a higher risk of developing heart disease. These findings underscore the urgent need to reduce our intake of processed foods and added sugars.

High-fructose corn syrup and refined carbohydrates are particularly insidious when it comes to promoting visceral fat and cardiovascular damage. Visceral fat is the fat that surrounds our internal organs, and it's strongly linked to an increased risk of heart disease. When we consume high-fructose corn syrup and refined carbohydrates, our bodies metabolize them differently than other types of sugars and carbs. This unique metabolism can lead to an increase in visceral fat, as well as other harmful substances like triglycerides and LDL cholesterol, both of which contribute to heart disease.

So, what can we do to protect ourselves and our families from these silent killers? The first step is to become savvy label readers. Learn to identify hidden sugars and artificial additives in the ingredients list. Next, make a plan to reduce your intake of processed foods and sugars gradually. This might involve meal planning and preparing more meals at home using whole, unprocessed ingredients. When cravings strike, reach for healthy alternatives like fresh fruits, nuts, or dark chocolate with a high cocoa content.

One of the most significant benefits of a whole-foods-based diet is its ability to help manage cravings and improve overall health. When we nourish our bodies with nutrient-dense, unprocessed foods, we're less likely to experience the blood sugar crashes that lead to intense cravings for sugary, processed snacks.

Moreover, a whole-foods-based diet provides our bodies with the essential nutrients they need to function optimally, reducing the risk of chronic diseases like heart disease.

It's essential to address some common misconceptions about processed foods and sugar. One such myth is that 'natural' sugars, like those found in honey or maple syrup, are healthier than refined sugars. While these natural sugars may contain some beneficial nutrients, they can still contribute to inflammation, insulin resistance, and other health problems when consumed in excess. Another misconception is that artificial sweeteners are a safe alternative to sugar. However, research has shown that artificial sweeteners can also contribute to poor health outcomes, including an increased risk of heart disease.

Consider the case of John, a 45-year-old man who was diagnosed with high blood pressure and prediabetes. John's diet was heavily reliant on processed foods and sugary snacks. With the guidance of a healthcare professional, John began to eliminate processed foods and added sugars from his diet, replacing them with whole, unprocessed foods. Within six months, John's blood pressure had normalized, and his blood sugar levels had significantly improved. His story is a testament to the power of dietary changes in improving heart health and overall well-being.

In conclusion, processed foods and sugars are indeed silent killers of the heart. By understanding the risks they pose and taking proactive steps to reduce our intake, we can significantly improve our heart health and overall well-being. Remember, every small change counts, and with time and consistency, you can take control of your health and protect your heart for years to come.

The Importance of Hydration and Electrolyte Balance for Circulation

In a world where our health is constantly under siege by processed foods, environmental toxins, and misleading information from centralized institutions, it's crucial to take control of our well-being. One of the most fundamental yet often overlooked aspects of heart health is proper hydration and electrolyte balance. Let's dive into why these elements are so vital for our cardiovascular system and how we can optimize them naturally.

Water is the essence of life, and our bodies are made up of about 60% water. It plays a crucial role in supporting cardiovascular function. Adequate hydration maintains blood volume, which is essential for circulation. When we're well-hydrated, our heart can pump blood more efficiently, delivering oxygen and nutrients to our cells and removing waste products. This process keeps our cells healthy and functioning optimally. Moreover, water helps regulate our body temperature and lubricates our joints, making physical activity more comfortable and beneficial for our heart health.

Dehydration, on the other hand, poses significant risks to our cardiovascular system. When we don't consume enough water, our blood becomes thicker and more viscous. This increased viscosity makes it harder for our heart to pump blood, reducing circulation and forcing our heart to work harder. Over time, this can lead to elevated blood pressure, a major risk factor for heart disease.

Furthermore, dehydration can cause an imbalance in electrolytes, which are essential for maintaining proper heart rhythm and function. It's alarming how such a simple aspect of our health can have such profound impacts, yet it's often ignored by mainstream medicine.

Electrolytes are minerals that carry an electric charge and are vital for various bodily functions, including heart health. The primary electrolytes are sodium, potassium, magnesium, and calcium. Sodium helps regulate blood pressure and volume, while potassium is crucial for maintaining a steady heartbeat. Magnesium plays a role in over 300 enzymatic reactions, including those involved in muscle and nerve function, which are essential for heart health. Calcium is necessary for muscle contractions, including the beating of our heart. An imbalance in any of these electrolytes can lead to irregular heartbeats, high blood pressure, and other cardiovascular issues.

Research has shown that proper hydration and electrolyte balance can significantly reduce the risk of heart disease and stroke. A study published in the Journal of the American College of Nutrition found that individuals who drank five or more glasses of water per day had a significantly lower risk of fatal coronary heart disease compared to those who drank two or fewer glasses. Another study in the British Medical Journal showed that adequate hydration can reduce the risk of stroke. These findings highlight the importance of something as simple as drinking enough water for our heart health.

Maintaining optimal hydration doesn't have to be complicated. A good rule of thumb is to drink half your body weight (in pounds in ounces of water daily. For example, if you weigh 150 pounds, aim for 75 ounces of water per day. However, this can vary based on your activity level, climate, and individual needs. It's essential to listen to your body and drink when you're thirsty. Signs of dehydration include dark yellow urine, fatigue, dizziness, and dry mouth. To maintain electrolyte balance, focus on a diet rich in fruits, vegetables, nuts, and seeds.

These foods provide a natural source of electrolytes without the added sugars and artificial ingredients found in many sports drinks.

Mineral-rich water and natural electrolytes can further support heart health. Mineral water contains essential minerals like calcium, magnesium, and potassium, which can contribute to your daily electrolyte needs. Natural electrolytes from foods like coconut water, bananas, and leafy greens can help maintain proper heart function and hydration. These natural sources are far superior to processed alternatives, which often contain harmful additives and artificial ingredients.

There are many misconceptions about hydration that can lead to confusion. One common myth is that all fluids are equally hydrating. In reality, beverages containing caffeine or alcohol can have a diuretic effect, increasing urine production and potentially leading to dehydration. Another misconception is that thirst is a reliable indicator of hydration status. By the time you feel thirsty, you may already be mildly dehydrated. It's important to sip water throughout the day rather than waiting until you're thirsty to drink.

Hydration is particularly important for managing chronic conditions like hypertension and heart failure. In individuals with hypertension, proper hydration can help maintain blood volume and pressure, reducing the strain on the heart.

For those with heart failure, adequate hydration can prevent the thickening of blood and reduce the risk of complications. It's a simple yet powerful tool in managing these conditions naturally, without relying solely on pharmaceutical interventions that often come with harmful side effects.

Let's consider the case of John, a 55-year-old man with a history of high blood pressure. Despite taking medication, John's blood pressure remained elevated, and he often felt fatigued. After learning about the importance of hydration, John decided to prioritize his water intake and focus on electrolyte-rich foods. He started drinking mineral water and incorporated more fruits, vegetables, and nuts into his diet. Within a few months, John noticed a significant improvement in his energy levels and a reduction in his blood pressure. His doctor was able to lower his medication dosage, and John felt more in control of his health. This case highlights the power of natural interventions and the importance of taking charge of our well-being.

In conclusion, proper hydration and electrolyte balance are fundamental yet often overlooked aspects of heart health. By understanding the role of water and electrolytes in our cardiovascular system, we can take simple yet powerful steps to support our heart health naturally. It's time to move beyond the misleading information from centralized institutions and embrace the power of natural medicine. Let's raise a glass of water to our heart health and the freedom to take control of our well-being.

REFERENCES:

- *No relevant citations found.*

How Gut Health Directly Impacts Cardiovascular Function

In an age where mainstream medicine often overlooks the profound connections within our bodies, it's crucial to understand how gut health directly impacts cardiovascular function. Let's embark on this journey together, exploring the intricate relationship between our gut and heart, and how nurturing one can significantly benefit the other.

At the core of this relationship is the gut microbiome, a bustling community of trillions of bacteria residing in our digestive system. Far from being mere bystanders, these microscopic inhabitants play a pivotal role in our overall health, particularly in inflammation and metabolism. When our gut microbiome is balanced and diverse, it helps regulate inflammation, a key factor in cardiovascular health. However, when this delicate balance is disrupted -- a condition known as gut dysbiosis -- it can lead to increased inflammation, oxidative stress, and endothelial dysfunction, all of which are significant risk factors for heart disease.

Gut dysbiosis is not just a digestive issue; it's a systemic problem that can have far-reaching consequences for our cardiovascular system. Increased inflammation, for instance, can damage the endothelial cells lining our blood vessels, leading to atherosclerosis -- a condition where plaques build up in the arteries, restricting blood flow and increasing the risk of heart attacks and strokes. Moreover, gut dysbiosis can impair our metabolism, leading to conditions like obesity, diabetes, and metabolic syndrome, all of which are closely linked to heart disease.

The mechanisms by which gut health influences heart health are fascinating and multifaceted. One of the key players in this process is short-chain fatty acids (SCFAs), which are produced when our gut bacteria ferment dietary fiber. SCFAs have been shown to have numerous beneficial effects on cardiovascular health, including reducing inflammation, improving endothelial function, and regulating blood pressure. Additionally, a healthy gut microbiome can help regulate our immune system, preventing it from overreacting and causing chronic inflammation that can damage our cardiovascular system.

Research has shed light on the specific gut bacteria that play a role in atherosclerosis and hypertension. For example, certain bacteria in our gut can produce trimethylamine N-oxide (TMAO), a compound that has been linked to an increased risk of atherosclerosis. On the other hand, other bacteria can produce beneficial compounds like SCFAs that help protect our cardiovascular system. By understanding these complex interactions, we can begin to appreciate the profound impact that our gut health has on our heart health.

The benefits of a healthy gut microbiome extend beyond just reducing the risk of heart disease. A balanced gut microbiome can also help improve our overall metabolic health, reducing the risk of obesity, diabetes, and metabolic syndrome. These conditions are not just risk factors for heart disease; they are also significant contributors to our overall health and well-being. By taking care of our gut health, we can address these conditions at their root, improving our overall health and reducing our reliance on mainstream medicine.

Improving gut health is not just about taking probiotics or eating yogurt. It's about making comprehensive lifestyle changes that support a diverse and balanced gut microbiome. This includes eating a diet rich in fiber and fermented foods, managing stress, and avoiding unnecessary antibiotics that can disrupt our gut microbiome. Additionally, it's crucial to be skeptical of mainstream medical advice that often overlooks the importance of gut health and instead pushes for pharmaceutical interventions that can have harmful side effects.

It's also important to address common misconceptions about gut health. Not all bacteria are harmful; in fact, most of the bacteria in our gut are beneficial and play crucial roles in our health. Moreover, probiotics are not just for digestive issues; they can have systemic benefits, including improving our cardiovascular health. By understanding these nuances, we can make informed decisions about our health and take control of our well-being.

Let's consider the case of a patient who improved their heart health by addressing gut dysbiosis. This individual, who had been struggling with high blood pressure and cholesterol, decided to take a natural approach to their health. They started by improving their diet, incorporating more fiber and fermented foods, and taking a high-quality probiotic. Over time, they noticed significant improvements in their blood pressure and cholesterol levels. Moreover, they felt more energetic and overall healthier. This case study highlights the profound impact that gut health can have on our cardiovascular health and the importance of taking a holistic approach to our well-being.

In conclusion, the connection between gut health and cardiovascular function is profound and multifaceted. By understanding and nurturing this relationship, we can take control of our health and reduce our reliance on mainstream medicine. It's time to embrace a more holistic and natural approach to our well-being, one that acknowledges the intricate connections within our bodies and the profound impact that our lifestyle choices can have on our health.

The Benefits of Fermented Foods for Heart Disease Prevention

For centuries, traditional cultures have understood something modern medicine is only now beginning to rediscover: fermented foods are not just delicious -- they're powerful medicine for the heart. Unlike the processed, chemical-laden foods pushed by corporate food giants, fermented foods are alive, teeming with beneficial microbes that restore balance to the gut and, in turn, protect the cardiovascular system. The pharmaceutical industry would rather you believe heart disease is a lifelong sentence requiring expensive statins or blood pressure pills, but the truth is far simpler -- and far more empowering. By embracing fermented foods, you're not just nourishing your body; you're reclaiming control over your health from a system that profits from keeping you sick.

Fermented foods are those that have undergone natural microbial transformation, breaking down sugars and starches into compounds that enhance digestion, nutrient absorption, and immune function. Think of them as nature's probiotics, but far more potent than any capsule you'd find in a drugstore.

Sauerkraut, kimchi, kefir, kombucha, and miso are among the most well-studied, each offering unique benefits for heart health. These foods work by populating the gut with diverse, beneficial bacteria that communicate directly with the cardiovascular system. When the gut microbiome is thriving, inflammation -- the silent driver of heart disease -- is kept in check. The gut-heart connection is so strong that researchers now refer to it as the 'gut-heart axis,' a relationship the pharmaceutical industry has conveniently ignored while pushing synthetic drugs with dangerous side effects.

One of the most compelling reasons to include fermented foods in your diet is their ability to reduce chronic inflammation, a root cause of atherosclerosis, high blood pressure, and metabolic syndrome. Studies have shown that the short-chain fatty acids (SCFAs) produced during fermentation -- such as butyrate, propionate, and acetate --

act as signaling molecules that regulate immune responses and lower inflammation throughout the body. For example, kimchi, a staple in Korean cuisine, has been found to improve lipid profiles by reducing LDL ('bad' cholesterol) and triglycerides while increasing HDL ('good' cholesterol). Similarly, kefir, a fermented dairy product, has been shown to lower blood pressure and reduce markers of oxidative stress, a key contributor to arterial damage. These are not fringe claims; they're findings from peer-reviewed research that mainstream medicine would rather suppress in favor of patented drugs.

But how exactly do these foods work their magic? The answer lies in their ability to modulate the gut microbiome, which in turn influences everything from blood pressure to cholesterol metabolism. When you consume fermented foods, the beneficial bacteria they contain -- such as Lactobacillus and Bifidobacterium --colonize the gut, crowding out harmful microbes that produce toxins linked to heart disease. These good bacteria also help metabolize dietary fiber into SCFAs, which have been shown to improve endothelial function (the health of blood vessel linings and reduce the risk of plaque buildup. Miso, for instance, contains enzymes that help break down proteins into bioactive peptides, some of which have been found to inhibit angiotensin-converting enzyme (ACE, a mechanism similar to that of blood pressure medications -- but without the side effects.

The benefits don't stop there. Fermented foods also enhance nutrient absorption, ensuring that the vitamins and minerals critical for heart health -- like magnesium, potassium, and B vitamins -- are more bioavailable. Kombucha, for example, is rich in B vitamins, which are essential for homocysteine metabolism; elevated homocysteine levels are a known risk factor for cardiovascular disease.

Sauerkraut, meanwhile, is packed with vitamin K2, a nutrient that directs calcium away from arteries (where it can cause dangerous plaques) and into bones (where it belongs). This is a stark contrast to the synthetic vitamins often recommended by doctors, which are poorly absorbed and sometimes even harmful in high doses.

If you're new to fermented foods, incorporating them into your diet is easier than you might think. Start with small servings -- perhaps a tablespoon of sauerkraut with lunch or a half-cup of kefir in the morning -- and gradually increase as your gut adjusts. For those who enjoy hands-on approaches, home fermentation is a rewarding and cost-effective way to take control of your food supply. Making sauerkraut, for instance, requires little more than cabbage, salt, and time.

Kombucha can be brewed at home with a SCOBY (symbiotic culture of bacteria and yeast, tea, and sugar), which the microbes consume during fermentation. The key is consistency; like any natural remedy, fermented foods work best when consumed regularly as part of a whole-foods diet.

It's also worth noting that fermented foods work synergistically with other gut-healthy practices. Pairing them with prebiotic foods -- like garlic, onions, and dandelion greens -- feeds the beneficial bacteria, amplifying their effects. Probiotic supplements can offer additional support, though they're no substitute for the complexity and diversity of microbes found in whole fermented foods. This holistic approach stands in sharp contrast to the reductionist model of modern medicine, which treats symptoms with isolated chemicals while ignoring the root causes of disease. By focusing on the gut, you're addressing the foundation of heart health, something no prescription drug can claim to do.

Despite the overwhelming evidence, there are still misconceptions about fermented foods. Some dismiss them as mere 'digestive aids,' failing to recognize their systemic benefits. Others assume they're difficult to prepare or unpalatable, not realizing that many fermented foods -- like miso soup or flavored kefir -- are delicious and versatile. Worst of all is the myth that fermented foods lack scientific backing, a narrative perpetuated by those who profit from keeping people dependent on pharmaceuticals. In reality, the research is robust and growing. A 2024 article from NaturalNews.com highlighted how traditional fermented foods like natto and tempeh have been used for centuries to support longevity and cardiovascular health, long before Big Pharma existed.

Consider the case of Mark, a 58-year-old man with a family history of heart disease. Despite taking statins for years, his cholesterol levels remained high, and he struggled with fatigue and brain fog. After learning about the gut-heart connection, he began incorporating kimchi, kefir, and homemade sauerkraut into his daily meals. Within three months, his LDL cholesterol dropped by 30 points, his blood pressure normalized, and his energy levels soared. His doctor was stunned -- so much so that he reluctantly admitted the dietary changes 'might be helping.' Mark's story isn't an outlier; it's a testament to what happens when we trust nature over synthetic solutions. The body has an incredible capacity to heal when given the right tools, and fermented foods are among the most powerful tools available.

In a world where the food supply is increasingly contaminated with pesticides, GMOs, and artificial additives, fermented foods offer a return to real, unadulterated nutrition. They're a reminder that true health doesn't come from a pill bottle or a government-approved diet plan. It comes from the earth, from traditions passed down through generations, and from the wisdom of our own bodies. By choosing fermented foods, you're not just preventing heart disease --you're taking a stand against a medical system that has failed millions. You're embracing a way of life that values self-reliance, natural healing, and the freedom to nourish yourself without interference from corporations or bureaucrats. And that, perhaps more than anything, is the ultimate act of heart health.

REFERENCES:

- NaturalNews.com. Top five traditional fermented anti aging foods - NaturalNews.com, May 28, 2024.

Understanding the Role of Fiber in Reducing Heart Disease Risk

When we talk about protecting our hearts, most people think of cutting out fatty foods or hitting the treadmill. But there's a quiet hero in the world of heart health that often gets overlooked -- fiber. Not the kind that keeps your internet running, but the kind that keeps your heart running smoothly. Fiber isn't just about keeping things moving in your digestive system; it's a powerhouse nutrient that can slash your risk of heart disease, lower your cholesterol, and even help manage your blood sugar. The best part? It's found in real, whole foods -- no prescription needed.

So, what exactly is fiber? Think of it as the indigestible part of plants that your body can't break down. But just because it passes through you doesn't mean it's not doing important work. Fiber comes in two main types: soluble and insoluble. Soluble fiber dissolves in water and forms a gel-like substance in your gut. This type is the superstar for heart health because it binds to cholesterol particles and helps escort them out of your body before they can clog your arteries. Foods like oats, apples, beans, and flaxseeds are packed with soluble fiber. Insoluble fiber, on the other hand, doesn't dissolve. It adds bulk to your stool and keeps your digestive system running like a well-oiled machine. You'll find it in foods like whole grains, nuts, and the skins of fruits and vegetables. Both types are essential, but when it comes to protecting your heart, soluble fiber is the real MVP.

Now, let's talk about how fiber actually works its magic. Imagine your bloodstream as a highway, and cholesterol as the traffic. Too much of the wrong kind of traffic -- like LDL cholesterol -- can cause a pileup in your arteries, leading to blockages and heart disease. Soluble fiber acts like a traffic cop, pulling excess LDL cholesterol out of circulation and sending it to your liver to be processed and removed. But that's not all. Fiber also helps regulate your blood sugar by slowing down how quickly your body absorbs sugar from your food. This keeps your insulin levels steady, which is crucial because high insulin levels can damage your arteries over time and increase your risk of heart disease. Plus, fiber keeps you feeling full longer, which helps you avoid overeating and the weight gain that often comes with it -- another big win for your heart.

The research on fiber and heart health is nothing short of impressive. Studies have consistently shown that people who eat more fiber have a lower risk of heart disease. For example, a large review of multiple studies found that for every additional 7 grams of fiber people ate per day, their risk of heart disease dropped by 9 percent. That's a big deal when you consider that most Americans only get about half the fiber they need -- around 15 grams a day instead of the recommended 25 to 38 grams. Fiber doesn't just lower LDL cholesterol; it also helps reduce blood pressure, another major risk factor for heart disease. And because fiber-rich foods are typically packed with other heart-healthy nutrients like antioxidants, vitamins, and minerals, you're giving your body a whole arsenal of protection with every bite.

So, where can you find this heart-protecting nutrient? The good news is, fiber is abundant in foods that are delicious and easy to incorporate into your meals. Start with fruits like berries, apples, and pears -- just be sure to eat the skins, where a lot of the fiber is hiding. Vegetables like broccoli, carrots, and Brussels sprouts are also fantastic sources. Legumes, such as lentils, chickpeas, and black beans, are fiber powerhouses and can be tossed into soups, salads, or even blended into dips like hummus. Whole grains like quinoa, brown rice, and oats are another great option, but be wary of processed "whole grain" products that might be loaded with added sugars or unhealthy fats. Nuts and seeds, including almonds, chia seeds, and flaxseeds, are not only high in fiber but also provide healthy fats that further support heart health.

If you're not used to eating a lot of fiber, it's best to increase your intake gradually. Jumping from 10 grams a day to 30 grams overnight can leave you feeling bloated or gassy -- your gut bacteria need time to adjust to the new fuel source. Start by adding one extra serving of fiber-rich food per day, like swapping white rice for brown rice or snacking on an apple instead of chips. Drink plenty of water, too, because fiber works best when it's well-hydrated. Over time, your digestive system will adapt, and you'll start reaping the benefits without the discomfort. Meal planning can make this transition easier. Try starting your day with a bowl of oatmeal topped with berries and flaxseeds, or whip up a big batch of vegetable and bean soup for lunches during the week. Small changes add up, and before you know it, you'll be hitting your fiber goals without even thinking about it.

Fiber isn't just a one-trick pony for heart health -- it also plays a crucial role in managing chronic conditions that are major risk factors for heart disease, like diabetes and obesity. For people with diabetes, fiber helps slow the absorption of sugar, preventing the spikes and crashes in blood sugar that can damage blood vessels over time. This steady blood sugar control is key to protecting your heart, as diabetes dramatically increases your risk of cardiovascular problems. Fiber also helps with weight management by promoting satiety, which means you're less likely to overeat or snack on unhealthy foods. Obesity is a well-known risk factor for heart disease, so keeping your weight in check with a fiber-rich diet is a smart strategy for long-term heart health.

There's a lot of misinformation out there about fiber, and it's important to set the record straight. One common myth is that all fiber supplements are created equal. The truth is, whole food sources of fiber are always superior because they come packaged with other beneficial nutrients that work synergistically to support your health. While supplements can be helpful in a pinch, they shouldn't be your primary source of fiber. Another misconception is that a high-fiber diet is bland or boring. Nothing could be further from the truth!

Fiber-rich foods are some of the most flavorful and versatile ingredients in the kitchen. Think about the rich, earthy taste of lentils in a spicy curry, the crunch of almonds in a salad, or the sweet juiciness of a ripe pear. Eating for heart health doesn't mean sacrificing taste -- it means discovering a whole new world of delicious, nourishing foods.

Let me share a story with you about a patient I'll call Mark. Mark came to me in his early 50s with high cholesterol, borderline high blood pressure, and a family history of heart disease. He was on the verge of being put on statins, but he wanted to try a natural approach first. We started by overhauling his diet to focus on fiber-rich foods. He swapped his morning cereal for steel-cut oats with berries, added a big salad with chickpeas to his lunch, and started snacking on nuts and seeds instead of crackers. Within three months, his LDL cholesterol dropped by 20 points, his blood pressure normalized, and he'd lost 10 pounds -- all without medication. Mark's story isn't unique. Time and again, I've seen how something as simple as increasing fiber intake can transform heart health. It's a reminder that sometimes, the most powerful medicine doesn't come in a pill -- it comes on your plate.

In a world where so much of our health advice is controlled by pharmaceutical companies and government agencies pushing expensive, synthetic solutions, it's empowering to know that something as natural and accessible as fiber can have such a profound impact on heart health. Fiber doesn't require a prescription, a doctor's visit, or a hefty price tag. It's a tool you can use every day to take control of your health, reduce your reliance on the medical system, and protect your heart for years to come. So next time you're at the grocery store, load up on those colorful fruits, crisp vegetables, hearty legumes, and crunchy nuts. Your heart will thank you -- one delicious, fiber-filled bite at a time.

Creating a Heart-Healthy Meal Plan for Long-Term Wellness

Imagine your heart as the engine of a well-oiled machine -- one that thrives on the right fuel, runs smoothly when cared for, and breaks down when neglected. The modern world, with its processed foods, synthetic additives, and pharmaceutical-driven health advice, has led millions down a path of chronic illness, particularly heart disease. But here's the truth: you don't need a prescription or a hospital stay to turn things around. Nature has already provided everything your heart needs to heal and thrive -- if you know where to look and how to use it.

A heart-healthy meal plan isn't just about cutting out the bad; it's about flooding your body with the good. Whole foods -- unprocessed, unrefined, and as close to their natural state as possible -- are the foundation. Think vibrant leafy greens, deep-colored berries, wild-caught fatty fish, raw nuts, and seeds. These foods are packed with fiber, which scrubs your arteries clean like a natural broom, sweeping out the plaque and toxins that clog your cardiovascular system. Healthy fats, like those found in avocados, olive oil, and coconut, don't just satisfy hunger -- they nourish your heart cells, reduce inflammation, and keep your blood flowing smoothly. And let's not forget the power of anti-inflammatory ingredients like turmeric, ginger, and garlic, which act like nature's fire extinguishers, cooling the chronic inflammation that's at the root of nearly every heart condition.

The benefits of this kind of eating go far beyond just preventing heart disease -- it can reverse it. Study after study has shown that a diet rich in whole, nutrient-dense foods improves lipid profiles, lowering harmful LDL cholesterol while boosting protective HDL. It reduces inflammation markers like C-reactive protein, which are strong predictors of heart attacks. It even enhances metabolic health, helping your body regulate blood sugar and insulin levels, which are deeply connected to heart function. When you eat this way, you're not just avoiding a heart attack; you're rebuilding a stronger, more resilient cardiovascular system from the inside out.

So how do you create a meal plan that works for you? Start by assessing your current habits -- honestly. What are you eating now? How does it make you feel? Energy levels, digestion, mood -- these are all clues. Next, set clear but flexible goals. Maybe you want to lower your blood pressure, reduce your reliance on medication, or simply have more energy to play with your kids. Then, stock your kitchen with the right tools: a good blender for smoothies, glass containers for meal prepping, and a well-organized pantry filled with staples like quinoa, lentils, and organic spices. Meal prepping doesn't have to be complicated -- cook a big batch of grains and roasted veggies on Sunday, and you've got the base for lunches and dinners all week.

Now, let's talk about the stars of the show -- the foods that should be front and center in your meal plan. Leafy greens like kale, spinach, and Swiss chard are packed with magnesium, a mineral that helps regulate heart rhythm and blood pressure. Fatty fish like wild salmon, sardines, and mackerel deliver omega-3s, which are like liquid gold for your heart, reducing triglycerides and preventing dangerous blood clots. Nuts and seeds -- walnuts, almonds, flaxseeds, chia -- are crunchy powerhouses of healthy fats, fiber, and plant sterols that actively lower cholesterol. Whole grains like steel-cut oats, brown rice, and farro provide steady energy without the blood sugar spikes that damage your arteries over time. And don't forget the herbs and spices: cinnamon to stabilize blood sugar, cayenne to improve circulation, and rosemary to protect your blood vessels.

Of course, it's just as important to know what to avoid. Processed foods are the enemy -- packaged with artificial ingredients, refined sugars, and industrial seed oils like soybean and canola, which are highly inflammatory and linked to heart disease. These foods are designed to be addictive, hijacking your taste buds and leaving you craving more while your heart pays the price. Even so-called "heart-healthy" products marketed by Big Food -- like low-fat yogurts loaded with sugar or margarine made from hydrogenated oils -- are wolves in sheep's clothing. Your best defense? Stick to the perimeter of the grocery store where the real food lives, and avoid anything with a long list of ingredients you can't pronounce.

One of the biggest myths is that eating for heart health means deprivation or bland meals. Nothing could be further from the truth. A heart-healthy plate is a feast for the senses -- colorful, flavorful, and deeply satisfying. For example, a Mediterranean-style breakfast might include a veggie omelet with spinach, tomatoes, and feta, drizzled with olive oil and served with a slice of whole-grain toast. Lunch could be a big salad with mixed greens, grilled salmon, avocado, and a lemon-tahini dressing. Dinner might feature grass-fed beef stir-fried with broccoli, mushrooms, and garlic, served over quinoa. Snacks? How about a handful of walnuts and dark chocolate, or hummus with crudités? The key is variety -- rotating your foods to ensure you're getting a broad spectrum of nutrients while keeping your taste buds excited.

But life isn't lived in a vacuum, and neither is your meal plan. Consistency matters, but so does flexibility. Dining out doesn't have to derail your progress -- just choose restaurants that prioritize fresh, whole ingredients, and don't be afraid to ask for substitutions. Cravings? They're normal, especially when transitioning away from processed foods. Instead of fighting them, satisfy them with healthier versions -- like frozen banana "nice cream" instead of ice cream, or air-popped popcorn with nutritional yeast instead of buttery microwave popcorn. The goal isn't perfection; it's progress. Some days will be easier than others, and that's okay. What matters is the long-term commitment to nourishing your heart.

Making this way of eating sustainable is all about integrating it into your lifestyle. Batch cooking saves time and ensures you always have healthy options on hand. Leftovers aren't just convenient -- they're a strategy. Double a recipe for dinner, and you've got lunch for the next day. Involve your family in the process, too. Kids are more likely to eat veggies they helped wash and chop, and partners who cook with you are more likely to stay on track. Gardening, even on a small scale, connects you to your food in a powerful way -- there's nothing like the taste of a tomato you grew yourself or the satisfaction of knowing exactly what went into it. Challenges will come up -- time constraints, budget concerns, social pressures --but they're not insurmountable. Time is often the biggest hurdle, but remember:

spending an hour on Sunday to prep meals saves you hours during the week. Budget-wise, whole foods can be affordable if you focus on seasonal produce, buy in bulk, and choose frozen organic veggies when fresh are too expensive. Social situations can be trickier, especially when friends or family don't share your health goals. Stand firm in your choices, but avoid preaching -- lead by example. When people see your energy, your glowing skin, and your vitality, they'll start asking for your secrets.

Let's look at a real-life example. Take Mark, a 52-year-old man who came to me after a scare with high blood pressure and chest pains. His doctor wanted to put him on statins and blood pressure medication for life. Instead, Mark committed to a heart-healthy meal plan rich in leafy greens, fatty fish, nuts, and seeds, while cutting out processed foods and sugar. Within three months, his blood pressure normalized, his cholesterol improved, and his energy levels soared. A year later, he was off all medication, running 5Ks, and had lost 20 pounds -- without ever feeling deprived. His story isn't unique; it's what happens when you give your body the tools it needs to heal itself.

The bottom line? Your heart doesn't need a pharmaceutical crutch -- it needs real food, the kind that's been sustaining humans for millennia before Big Pharma and Big Food hijacked our plates. This isn't about following a rigid diet; it's about reclaiming your health, one meal at a time. When you eat this way, you're not just preventing heart disease -- you're building a body that's resilient, vibrant, and free from the shackles of the sick-care system. And that's a freedom worth fighting for.

5: Empowering Yourself Against Heart Disease

Imagine walking into a doctor's office and being handed a prescription without a single explanation -- no discussion of side effects, no mention of alternatives, not even a clear reason why this particular drug was chosen for you. For decades, this has been the norm in conventional medicine: a one-size-fits-all approach where patients are passive recipients of care rather than active participants in their own healing. But what if you could flip that script? What if you, not a white-coat authority or a pharmaceutical brochure, held the power to decide what goes into your body and how you heal? That's the promise of informed decision-making -- a radical act of reclaiming control over your heart health and your life.

Informed decision-making means gathering knowledge, questioning assumptions, and choosing your path with eyes wide open. It's not about rejecting modern medicine outright; it's about demanding transparency, weighing risks honestly, and refusing to outsource your well-being to institutions that have repeatedly prioritized profits over people. The stakes couldn't be higher. Heart disease remains the leading killer in the Western world, yet the solutions peddled by mainstream medicine -- statins, blood thinners, and invasive procedures --often come with devastating side effects and little proof they address the root causes of the problem. Meanwhile, natural therapies like magnesium supplementation, CoQ10, and dietary changes have been shown to reverse arterial plaque, lower blood pressure, and even repair damaged heart tissue --without the risks of pharmaceuticals. The choice seems obvious, but only if you're equipped to see through the noise.

Education is your first line of defense. The medical-industrial complex thrives on keeping patients in the dark, using jargon, fear, and false urgency to rush people into treatments they don't fully understand. But knowledge dismantles that control. Start by questioning everything: Why is cholesterol -- an essential substance your body produces -- suddenly labeled a villain? Why are statins prescribed to millions when studies show they offer negligible benefits for most people and increase the risk of diabetes and muscle wasting? Why are simple, low-cost interventions like vitamin K2 (which directs calcium into bones instead of arteries) or ground flaxseed (a natural blood thinner) rarely mentioned in cardiology offices? The answers often lead back to one uncomfortable truth: there's no profit in prevention or natural cures. Your job is to dig deeper. Seek out independent researchers, functional medicine practitioners, and patient testimonials from those who've reversed heart disease without drugs or surgery.

The more you learn, the harder it becomes for anyone to manipulate your choices.

Critical thinking is the next step. Not all information is created equal, and the internet is flooded with both life-saving wisdom and dangerous misinformation. How do you tell the difference? First, follow the money. If a source is funded by pharmaceutical companies or government agencies with ties to Big Pharma (like the FDA or NIH), approach it with skepticism. Second, look for censorship.

Platforms that silence dissent -- whether it's doctors questioning vaccine safety or nutritionists exposing the harms of seed oils -- are often protecting narratives, not health. Third, prioritize real-world outcomes over lab-coated theories. Does a treatment actually help people feel better and live longer, or does it just lower a number on a blood test while causing new problems? For example, statins might reduce LDL cholesterol, but if they also deplete CoQ10 (a nutrient critical for heart muscle function), are they really a net gain? Asking these questions isn't paranoia; it's due diligence.

Being an active participant in your health isn't just about better outcomes -- it's about reclaiming your dignity. Study after study shows that patients who engage in shared decision-making with their providers experience less anxiety, fewer complications, and higher satisfaction with their care. But why stop at shared decision-making? True empowerment means taking the lead. It means walking into a doctor's office with a list of questions: What are the alternatives to this drug? What lifestyle changes could achieve the same result? What are the long-term consequences of this procedure? It means refusing to accept "because I said so" as an answer. When you shift from passive compliance to informed consent, something profound happens: you stop being a victim of the system and start becoming its most formidable challenger. And that's when real healing begins.

So how do you put this into practice? Start by researching every recommendation before saying yes. If your doctor suggests a statin, ask for the data on its effectiveness for someone with your specific risk factors. (Spoiler: for many, the benefit is statistically insignificant.) If a stent is recommended, investigate whether enhanced external counterpulsation (EECP), a non-invasive therapy, could achieve the same goal without surgery. Seek second opinions -- not just from another conventional cardiologist, but from integrative or functional medicine practitioners who view the body as a whole system, not a collection of symptoms to suppress. And never underestimate the power of lifestyle. A plant-based, nutrient-dense diet, regular movement, and stress management have been proven to reverse coronary artery disease in studies like Dr. Dean Ornish's landmark research. Yet how many cardiologists prescribe kale instead of Lipitor?

The gap between what's profitable and what's effective is where your power lies.

Understanding risks and benefits is where many people get tripped up. Conventional medicine excels at framing its interventions as "safe and effective," but those terms are often misleading. A drug might be "safe" in the short term but cause irreversible damage over years. A procedure might be "effective" at unclogging an artery but do nothing to prevent new blockages from forming.

Natural therapies, on the other hand, are frequently dismissed as "unproven" --even when they've been used successfully for centuries. Take hawthorn berry, for example. This herb has been shown in multiple studies to improve heart function, reduce angina, and lower blood pressure, with virtually no side effects. Yet you'll rarely hear about it in a cardiologist's office because it can't be patented. The same goes for magnesium, which relaxes blood vessels, prevents arrhythmias, and reduces the risk of sudden cardiac death. These aren't fringe ideas; they're well-documented facts suppressed by a system that benefits from keeping you dependent.

Of course, barriers exist. Misinformation is rampant, and fear is a powerful tool used to keep people compliant. You might worry that stepping outside the conventional model will leave you without support or that natural approaches won't be "strong enough." But consider this: the most common cause of death in hospitals isn't heart attacks -- it's medical errors and adverse drug reactions. The system designed to "save" you is often the greatest threat to your survival. Lack of access to resources is another hurdle, but here's the good news: some of the most potent heart-healing tools are free or low-cost. Sunlight (for vitamin D), deep breathing (to activate the parasympathetic nervous system), and walking barefoot on grass (to reduce inflammation via grounding) don't require a prescription or insurance approval. And if you're overwhelmed, you're not alone. Patient advocacy groups and online communities -- like those at the Weston A. Price Foundation or the National Health Federation -- offer guidance, shared experiences, and even legal support for those challenging medical dogma.

Let's talk about what happens when you take control. Take the case of Robert, a 58-year-old man diagnosed with severe coronary artery disease. His cardiologist urged immediate bypass surgery, warning that without it, Robert was a "ticking time bomb." But Robert did his homework. He learned that bypass surgery often fails to extend life expectancy for stable patients and can lead to cognitive decline due to the heart-lung machine. Instead, he adopted a whole-food, plant-based diet rich in nitrates (from beets and leafy greens), started daily magnesium and CoQ10 supplementation, and incorporated stress-reduction techniques like meditation. Within months, his angina disappeared. A follow-up scan showed his arterial blockages had reduced by 20%. Five years later, he's still thriving -- without surgery or drugs. Robert's story isn't an outlier; it's a testament to what's possible when you refuse to accept the default path.

The choice is yours: will you hand over your health to a system that treats symptoms while ignoring causes, or will you become the CEO of your own well-being? Informed decision-making isn't just a strategy -- it's an act of rebellion against a medical establishment that has betrayed its oath to "first, do no harm." It's a declaration that your body belongs to you, not to pharmaceutical companies, not to insurance algorithms, and not to fear-mongering guidelines written by conflicted "experts." The tools are at your fingertips -- ancient herbs, cutting-edge nutrition science, and the unshakable knowledge that your body is designed to heal. All that's left is to decide: will you be a passive patient or an empowered healer? Your heart is waiting for your answer.

Building a Personalized Heart Health Plan for Life

In a world where mainstream medicine often overlooks the power of natural health and personal liberty, taking charge of your heart health is not just wise --it's essential. A personalized heart health plan is your roadmap to long-term cardiovascular wellness, tailored to your unique needs and lifestyle. It's about more than just avoiding heart disease; it's about thriving in a way that aligns with your body's natural rhythms and your personal values. By focusing on natural medicine, nutrition, and self-reliance, you can create a plan that truly serves your well-being without relying on the flawed systems of conventional healthcare.

A robust heart health plan is built on several key components, each playing a vital role in maintaining cardiovascular wellness. Nutrition is the foundation -- whole, organic foods rich in vitamins, minerals, and phytonutrients nourish your body and protect your heart. Exercise, particularly activities that you enjoy and can sustain, keeps your heart strong and resilient. Stress management, through practices like meditation, herbal remedies, or simply spending time in nature, helps to reduce the burden on your heart. Quality sleep is non-negotiable, as it allows your body to repair and regenerate. Lastly, reducing your exposure to toxins -- whether from processed foods, environmental pollutants, or harmful personal care products -- is crucial for long-term heart health. Each of these components works together to create a holistic approach to wellness that respects your body's natural processes.

Creating your personalized heart health plan begins with assessing your individual risk factors. This isn't about relying on mainstream medical assessments that often push unnecessary pharmaceuticals. Instead, consider your family history, current lifestyle, and any existing health conditions. From there, set clear, achievable goals that align with your values -- perhaps growing your own organic garden, incorporating more herbal remedies, or committing to daily walks in nature. Tracking your progress is equally important, not just through conventional metrics like blood pressure, but also through how you feel -- your energy levels, mental clarity, and overall well-being. This self-awareness is a powerful tool in natural health, allowing you to adjust your plan as needed without dependence on external authorities.

Flexibility and adaptability are at the heart of a sustainable heart health plan. Life is unpredictable, and your plan should be able to bend without breaking. If you encounter setbacks -- like a busy week that disrupts your routine or an unexpected stressor -- view them as opportunities to refine your approach rather than reasons to give up. Perhaps you need to adjust your exercise routine or find new ways to manage stress. The key is to stay committed to your overall vision of health while allowing room for life's inevitable changes. This adaptability is a cornerstone of self-reliance, ensuring that your plan remains effective and relevant to your life.

You don't have to go it alone. While personal liberty and self-reliance are crucial, having a support network can make all the difference. Seek out healthcare providers who respect natural medicine and your personal values -- those who will work with you rather than dictate to you. Coaches, particularly those who specialize in natural health, can offer guidance and motivation. Support networks, whether friends, family, or like-minded communities, provide encouragement and accountability. These relationships can help you stay on track, especially when facing challenges, and remind you that you're part of a larger movement toward decentralized, natural health.

Let's consider a few examples of personalized heart health plans tailored to different risk profiles. If you have hypertension, your plan might focus on a diet rich in potassium and magnesium, regular gentle exercise like yoga or swimming, and stress management through herbal teas and meditation. For someone with diabetes, the emphasis might be on a low-glycemic, whole-food diet, daily walks, and careful monitoring of blood sugar levels using natural methods. If heart disease runs in your family, your plan could include a strong focus on antioxidant-rich foods, regular detoxification practices, and stress reduction techniques. Each plan is as unique as the individual, reflecting their specific needs and circumstances while staying true to the principles of natural health.

Staying motivated and accountable is often the biggest challenge in maintaining a heart health plan. Journaling can be a powerful tool -- tracking not just what you eat or how much you exercise, but also how you feel and what you're grateful for each day. There are also apps designed to support natural health goals, helping you monitor progress and stay connected to your why. Celebrating milestones, no matter how small, reinforces your commitment and keeps you motivated.

Whether it's treating yourself to a relaxing herbal bath or sharing your success with your support network, these celebrations are vital to sustaining your journey.

Of course, challenges will arise. Time constraints, lack of support, and plateaus are common, but they're not insurmountable. If time is an issue, look for ways to integrate heart-healthy habits into your daily routine -- like growing a small herb garden or taking short, mindful walks during breaks. If you lack support, seek out communities, either locally or online, that share your values and can offer encouragement. Plateaus can be frustrating, but they're also an opportunity to reassess and refine your plan. Perhaps it's time to try a new herbal remedy, adjust your diet, or explore a different form of exercise. Each challenge is a chance to deepen your commitment to your health and your personal liberty.

Consider the case of a patient who built and maintained a personalized heart health plan for life. This individual, faced with a family history of heart disease, decided to take control of their health through natural means. They started an organic garden, incorporated daily walks in nature, and focused on a diet rich in whole, unprocessed foods. They also worked with a natural health coach to manage stress through meditation and herbal remedies. Over time, they not only improved their cardiovascular health but also inspired their family and community to embrace a more natural, self-reliant approach to wellness. Their journey is a testament to the power of personal liberty, natural medicine, and the human spirit's capacity for resilience and transformation.

Building a personalized heart health plan for life is more than just a series of steps -- it's a commitment to yourself, your values, and your well-being. It's about rejecting the one-size-fits-all approach of mainstream medicine and embracing a path that honors your unique needs and circumstances. By focusing on natural health, personal liberty, and self-reliance, you're not just preventing heart disease; you're creating a life of vitality, freedom, and empowerment. This is your journey, and it's one that can inspire others to take charge of their health in a way that aligns with their deepest values and beliefs.

The Importance of Regular Health Monitoring and Self-Assessment

In a world where our health is constantly under siege by processed foods, environmental toxins, and a medical system that often prioritizes profits over people, taking charge of our own well-being is not just empowering -- it's essential. Regular health monitoring and self-assessment are powerful tools in the fight against heart disease, a condition that mainstream medicine often mismanages with expensive, harmful drugs and procedures. By understanding and tracking key health metrics, we can make informed decisions that align with natural, holistic approaches to health. This section will guide you through the importance of health monitoring, the key metrics to track, and how to use this information to protect and improve your heart health naturally.

Health monitoring involves regularly checking and recording various aspects of your health, such as blood pressure, blood sugar levels, and heart rate variability. Self-assessment goes a step further, encouraging you to reflect on lifestyle factors like stress, sleep quality, and diet that might be impacting your heart health.

Together, these practices form a proactive approach to health that can help you detect potential issues early and make necessary adjustments before they become serious problems. Unlike the reactive nature of conventional medicine, which often waits until symptoms are severe before intervening with pharmaceuticals or surgeries, self-monitoring empowers you to take control of your health journey.

When it comes to heart health, several key metrics should be on your radar. Blood pressure is one of the most critical indicators. High blood pressure, or hypertension, is often called the 'silent killer' because it can damage your arteries and heart without causing noticeable symptoms. Monitoring your blood pressure at home with a simple, affordable device can help you catch potential issues early. Lipid profiles, which measure levels of cholesterol and triglycerides in your blood, are another important metric. However, it's crucial to understand that cholesterol is not the villain it's often made out to be by mainstream medicine. Instead of relying solely on pharmaceuticals to lower cholesterol, consider natural approaches like improving your diet and incorporating heart-healthy herbs and superfoods.

Blood sugar levels and inflammation markers are also vital to track. Chronic high blood sugar can lead to diabetes, a significant risk factor for heart disease.

Inflammation, often measured through markers like C-reactive protein, is another silent contributor to heart disease that mainstream medicine frequently overlooks. Heart rate variability, or HRV, is a newer metric gaining attention for its ability to reflect the balance of your autonomic nervous system. A higher HRV generally indicates better cardiovascular fitness and resilience to stress. By monitoring these metrics, you can gain a comprehensive view of your heart health and make informed decisions about your lifestyle and natural health strategies.

Monitoring these metrics at home has never been easier, thanks to advancements in technology and the availability of affordable, user-friendly devices. Wearable devices, like fitness trackers and smart-watches, can continuously monitor your heart rate, activity levels, and even HRV. Home testing kits are available for checking blood pressure, blood sugar, and lipid profiles. Regular check-ups with a healthcare provider who respects natural, holistic approaches can also be valuable, but remember that you are ultimately in charge of your health journey. Don't be afraid to seek second opinions or explore alternative therapies if something doesn't feel right.

The benefits of regular health monitoring are immense. Early detection of potential issues allows you to take action before problems become severe. Tracking your progress toward heart health goals can be incredibly motivating, showing you the tangible results of your efforts to improve your diet, increase your activity levels, or manage stress. Regular monitoring also provides valuable information that can help you and your healthcare provider make informed decisions about your health. For example, if you notice that your blood pressure is consistently high, you might decide to incorporate more potassium-rich foods, like bananas and leafy greens, or herbs known for their blood pressure-lowering effects, like hibiscus and garlic.

Self-assessment is equally important, as it encourages you to look beyond the numbers and consider how various lifestyle factors might be impacting your heart health. Stress, for instance, is a significant contributor to heart disease that is often overlooked by conventional medicine. By regularly assessing your stress levels and implementing natural stress-management techniques, like meditation, deep breathing, or spending time in nature, you can significantly improve your heart health. Sleep is another critical factor. Poor sleep quality or insufficient sleep can contribute to high blood pressure, inflammation, and weight gain -- all risk factors for heart disease. Diet, of course, is one of the most powerful tools we have for preventing and reversing heart disease. Regularly assessing your diet and making adjustments to include more whole, nutrient-dense foods can have a profound impact on your heart health.

Consider the story of John, a 55-year-old man who was told by his doctor that he needed to start taking statins for his high cholesterol. Uncomfortable with the idea of taking a pharmaceutical drug long-term, John decided to take a more natural approach. He began monitoring his blood pressure, blood sugar, and lipid profiles at home. He also started tracking his diet, stress levels, and sleep quality. Over time, John noticed that his cholesterol levels improved when he incorporated more soluble fiber, like oats and beans, and heart-healthy fats, like those found in avocados and nuts, into his diet. He also found that his blood pressure was lower on days when he practiced meditation and got a full night's sleep. Armed with this information, John was able to work with a healthcare provider who supported his natural approach and avoid the need for statins altogether.

Despite the clear benefits of regular health monitoring, there are common barriers that can make it challenging. Cost is one of the most significant. While some home testing devices and wearable technology can be expensive, there are often more affordable alternatives available. For example, manual blood pressure monitors are typically less expensive than automatic ones. Additionally, some insurance plans may cover the cost of certain devices or tests. Access to testing can also be a challenge, particularly for those living in rural or underserved areas. However, the growing popularity of telemedicine and home testing kits is making health monitoring more accessible than ever before. Fear of results is another common barrier. It's natural to feel anxious about what health monitoring might reveal, but remember that knowledge is power. The sooner you detect potential issues, the sooner you can take action to address them naturally.

Working with a healthcare provider who respects your desire for a natural, holistic approach to health is crucial. While home monitoring and self-assessment provide valuable information, a knowledgeable healthcare provider can help you interpret your results and make informed decisions about next steps. Don't be afraid to seek out providers who are open to alternative therapies and who will support your desire to take a proactive, natural approach to your health. Remember, you are the ultimate authority on your body and your health journey. By combining regular health monitoring, self-assessment, and the guidance of a trusted healthcare provider, you can take control of your heart health and protect yourself from the often harmful, profit-driven approaches of mainstream medicine.

In conclusion, regular health monitoring and self-assessment are powerful tools in the fight against heart disease. By understanding and tracking key health metrics, reflecting on lifestyle factors, and working with a supportive healthcare provider, you can take a proactive, natural approach to your heart health. Don't wait for mainstream medicine to tell you there's a problem -- take charge of your health journey today and empower yourself against heart disease naturally.

Overcoming Fear and Anxiety About Heart Disease with Knowledge

Fear and anxiety are natural responses to the unknown, but when it comes to heart disease, these emotions can become overwhelming and even harmful. Fear, in this context, is often a reaction to the perceived threat of heart disease, while anxiety is the persistent worry about the possibility of developing it or the consequences it may bring. Both emotions can have a significant impact on your cardiovascular health, creating a vicious cycle that exacerbates the very condition you fear. The good news is that knowledge is a powerful tool that can help you break free from this cycle, empowering you to take control of your heart health and overall well-being.

When you experience fear and anxiety, your body responds by releasing stress hormones like cortisol. While these hormones are essential for short-term survival situations, chronic elevation can lead to a host of problems. High cortisol levels can increase blood pressure, blood sugar, and cholesterol, all of which are risk factors for heart disease. Moreover, stress hormones can trigger inflammation, a key player in the development and progression of cardiovascular disease.

Inflammation can damage your blood vessels, making them more susceptible to the buildup of plaque, which can lead to heart attacks and strokes. Fear and anxiety can also lead to poor health behaviors, further increasing your risk of heart disease. When you're feeling stressed or anxious, you might be more likely to reach for comfort foods high in sugar and unhealthy fats, skip workouts, or have trouble sleeping. These behaviors can contribute to weight gain, high blood pressure, and other risk factors for heart disease. Additionally, stress can make it harder to stick to healthy habits, creating a negative feedback loop that can feel impossible to break.

One of the most effective ways to combat fear and anxiety about heart disease is through education. Understanding the true causes of heart disease and the power of natural prevention strategies can help you feel more in control of your health.

For instance, learning about the role of inflammation in heart disease can empower you to make dietary changes that reduce inflammation, such as eating more fruits, vegetables, and omega-3 fatty acids. Similarly, understanding the impact of stress on your heart can motivate you to prioritize stress management techniques like mindfulness and meditation.

Mindfulness is a practice that involves focusing your attention on the present moment, acknowledging and accepting your feelings, thoughts, and bodily sensations. It has been shown to reduce stress, lower blood pressure, and improve overall well-being. Cognitive-behavioral techniques, such as cognitive restructuring, can also help you challenge and change negative thought patterns that contribute to anxiety. Additionally, stress management strategies like deep breathing, yoga, and regular exercise can help you build resilience against the physical and emotional toll of stress.

Rather than letting fear control you, try reframing it as motivation for positive change. For example, if you're worried about your family history of heart disease, use that concern as a catalyst to adopt a heart-healthy lifestyle. This might include eating a nutrient-dense diet, engaging in regular physical activity, and prioritizing stress management. Similarly, if you're anxious about the possibility of a heart attack, let that anxiety drive you to seek support from loved ones, healthcare providers, or support groups. Remember, knowledge is power, and every step you take towards understanding and improving your heart health is a step away from fear and anxiety.

Research has shown a clear link between fear, anxiety, and heart disease. In fact, there's even a term for the excessive worry about heart-related sensations and the misinterpretation of bodily symptoms as signs of heart disease: cardiac anxiety.

This condition can lead to increased healthcare utilization, decreased quality of life, and even poorer recovery outcomes after a cardiac event. By understanding the connection between your emotions and your heart health, you can take proactive steps to manage your mental well-being and, in turn, support your cardiovascular health.

Common sources of fear and anxiety about heart disease include misinformation, personal or family history, and media portrayals. It's essential to address these sources head-on. For instance, if you're concerned about your family history, talk to your healthcare provider about your specific risks and what you can do to mitigate them. If you're feeling overwhelmed by media stories, limit your exposure and focus on reputable sources of information. And if you're struggling with misinformation, seek out evidence-based resources that can help you separate fact from fiction.

Building a support network is crucial for managing fear and anxiety about heart disease. This network can include healthcare providers, family, friends, and even support groups for people with similar concerns. Don't be afraid to lean on these individuals for emotional support, practical advice, and encouragement.

Remember, you don't have to face your fears alone. There are people who care about you and want to help you navigate this journey towards better heart health.

Consider the case of John, a 45-year-old man with a family history of heart disease. John was constantly worried about his heart health, leading to high stress levels and poor health behaviors. However, after attending a series of educational workshops on heart disease prevention, he began to understand the true causes of the condition and the power of natural prevention strategies. Armed with this knowledge, John started making positive changes in his life. He adopted a heart-healthy diet, began exercising regularly, and practiced mindfulness to manage his stress. Over time, John's fear and anxiety about heart disease decreased significantly. He felt more in control of his health and more optimistic about his future. John's story is a testament to the power of knowledge and the importance of taking an active role in your heart health journey.

In conclusion, fear and anxiety about heart disease are common, but they don't have to control your life. By understanding the impact of these emotions on your cardiovascular health, educating yourself about the true causes of heart disease, and taking proactive steps to manage your mental well-being, you can break free from the cycle of fear and anxiety. Remember, knowledge is power, and every step you take towards understanding and improving your heart health is a step towards a healthier, happier you.

The Role of Financial Independence in Accessing Natural Health Solutions

Imagine waking up every morning with the freedom to choose the best foods for your heart, the ability to visit a holistic practitioner without stressing over the bill, or the confidence to know that if illness strikes, you have the resources to heal naturally -- without being forced into a system that profits from your suffering.

This is the power of financial independence when it comes to natural health. But here's the hard truth: our current system is rigged to keep you dependent -- on processed foods, on pharmaceuticals, on a medical industry that thrives on repeat customers, not cures. Breaking free from that cycle isn't just about money; it's about reclaiming control over your body, your choices, and your future.

Financial independence, in the context of natural health, means having the resources to opt out of the industrialized sickness system. It's the ability to afford organic, nutrient-dense foods instead of chemically laden processed junk. It's the freedom to invest in high-quality supplements -- like magnesium for heart rhythm, CoQ10 for energy, or medicinal mushrooms for immunity -- without worrying about whether your insurance will cover them (spoiler: they won't. It's the security of knowing you can pay out-of-pocket for a functional medicine doctor who will actually listen to you, instead of being rushed through a 10-minute appointment with a physician who's incentivized to prescribe statins. Most importantly, it's the peace of mind that comes from not being financially bullied into choices that harm your long-term health.

The barriers to natural health are steep, and they're deliberately constructed. Organic foods can cost up to 50 percent more than conventional ones, not because they're inherently expensive to produce, but because the industrial food system is subsidized by taxpayer dollars funneled into Big Agra's pockets.

Supplements, even basic ones like vitamin D or omega-3s, are often treated as luxury items rather than the essential nutrients they are. And alternative therapies -- acupuncture, ozone therapy, or even something as simple as sauna sessions for detox -- are almost never covered by insurance. Why? Because the system isn't designed to keep you well; it's designed to keep you coming back for more pills, more procedures, and more profit-driven interventions. The message is clear: if you want to heal naturally, you'd better be prepared to pay for it yourself.

But here's what the fear-mongers won't tell you: investing in natural health is one of the smartest financial decisions you can make. Yes, a bottle of organic cold-pressed olive oil costs more upfront than a jug of vegetable oil laced with hexane. But that olive oil is protecting your arteries from inflammation, reducing your risk of heart disease, and saving you thousands in future medical bills. A $50 bottle of high-quality curcumin might seem pricey until you realize it's helping reverse endothelial dysfunction -- the same issue that would otherwise land you in a cardiologist's office facing a $30,000 stent procedure. The data is undeniable: people who prioritize preventive care spend far less on healthcare over their lifetimes. They miss fewer days of work, enjoy higher productivity, and -- most importantly -- avoid the financial and emotional devastation of chronic illness. Natural health isn't an expense; it's an investment with compounding returns. So how do you break free? It starts with rejecting the lie that you're powerless.

Financial independence in health isn't about being a millionaire; it's about reallocating resources toward what truly matters. Grow a garden -- even a small one -- and you've just cut your grocery bill while boosting your nutrient intake. Learn to ferment foods, and you're saving money on probiotics while improving gut health, which is directly linked to heart health. Invest in a quality water filter instead of bottled water, and you're avoiding endocrine-disrupting plastics while protecting your cardiovascular system. Every dollar you spend on these things is a dollar not spent on a future prescription or hospital stay.

Self-reliance is the ultimate rebellion against a system that wants you dependent. When you know how to grow your own food, you're no longer at the mercy of rising grocery prices or supply chain disruptions. When you understand basic herbal medicine -- like how hawthorn berry supports heart function or how garlic lowers blood pressure -- you're less likely to be strong-armed into pharmaceuticals with dangerous side effects. When you prioritize movement, sunlight, and stress management, you're reducing your reliance on a healthcare system that treats symptoms but rarely addresses root causes. This isn't just about saving money; it's about reclaiming sovereignty over your body and your life.

Let's talk about the elephant in the room: the myth that natural health is only for the wealthy. This is a deliberate distraction. The truth is, the real luxury is being able to afford the long-term consequences of poor health. A family eating fast food four times a week might save $20 today, but they're signing up for diabetes, obesity, and heart disease -- conditions that will drain their finances for decades.

On the other hand, someone who spends $100 a month on organic vegetables, grass-fed meat, and a few key supplements is making a down payment on a future free from medical debt. The system wants you to believe you can't afford to be healthy, but the reality is, you can't afford not to be.

Prioritizing health in your financial planning isn't optional; it's essential. This means setting aside funds for preventive care -- whether that's a yearly visit to a naturopath, a high-quality multivitamin, or a sauna for detox. It means viewing your health spending as non-negotiable, just like your mortgage or utilities. And it means recognizing that every dollar you invest in your well-being today is a dollar you won't lose to a medical emergency tomorrow. If you're not already budgeting for your health, start small: redirect $20 a week from a non-essential expense (like streaming services or takeout toward organic produce or a supplement. Over time, those small choices add up to massive savings -- and a heart that keeps beating strong.

Consider the story of Mark, a 52-year-old man who was told by his cardiologist that he needed statins and blood pressure medication for the rest of his life. Instead of accepting this sentence, Mark took control. He started a side business selling homegrown microgreens, which not only provided him with the most nutrient-dense foods on the planet but also generated extra income. He invested in a small freezer to buy grass-fed beef in bulk, saving money while flooding his body with heart-healthy fats. He traded his gym membership for a set of resistance bands and a rebounder, eliminating monthly fees while improving his circulation. Within a year, his blood pressure normalized, his cholesterol improved, and he'd cut his healthcare costs by 70 percent. Mark's story isn't unique -- it's a blueprint. Financial independence in health isn't about having endless resources; it's about using the resources you do have wisely, creatively, and with unwavering commitment to your well-being.

The path to natural health isn't paved with insurance claims or government handouts; it's built on personal responsibility, smart choices, and the courage to opt out of a broken system. It's about recognizing that your health is your most valuable asset -- and that no one will protect it as fiercely as you will. The tools are there: real food, time-tested herbs, movement, sunlight, clean water. The only question is whether you'll let financial barriers stand in your way or whether you'll take the steps -- however small -- to reclaim your power. Because when it comes to your heart, your freedom, and your future, the cost of inaction is always higher than the price of taking control.

Creating a Sustainable Lifestyle That Supports Heart Health

Creating a sustainable lifestyle that supports heart health is about making choices that you can maintain over the long term, choices that nourish your body, mind, and spirit. It's not about quick fixes or extreme measures that leave you feeling deprived or overwhelmed. Instead, it's about finding a balance that works for you, a balance that supports your heart health and overall well-being. A sustainable lifestyle is one that you can stick with, not just for a few weeks or months, but for years to come. It's about making changes that become habits, habits that become a natural part of your daily routine. This is important because heart health is not a short-term goal. It's a lifelong journey. The choices you make every day, from what you eat to how you manage stress, all add up to support or hinder your heart health. By creating a sustainable lifestyle, you're investing in your long-term well-being.

When it comes to the key components of a sustainable lifestyle, there are several areas to focus on. First, there's nutrition. This means eating a diet rich in whole, unprocessed foods, foods that are as close to their natural state as possible. Think fruits, vegetables, whole grains, lean proteins, and healthy fats. These foods provide the nutrients your body needs to function at its best, supporting heart health and overall well-being. Next, there's exercise. Regular physical activity is crucial for heart health. It helps strengthen your heart muscle, improves circulation, and can even help lower blood pressure. But exercise doesn't have to mean spending hours at the gym. It can be as simple as a daily walk, a dance class, or even gardening. The key is to find activities you enjoy and can stick with over the long term. Stress management is another important component. Chronic stress can take a toll on your heart health, so finding ways to manage stress is essential. This could be through meditation, deep breathing, yoga, or any other practice that helps you relax and unwind. Sleep is also vital. Quality sleep allows your body to rest and repair, supporting overall health, including heart health.

Lastly, reducing your exposure to toxins is important. This means choosing natural, non-toxic products for your home and body, as well as being mindful of environmental toxins.

Creating a sustainable lifestyle is all about practical strategies that you can incorporate into your daily life. Start by setting realistic goals. Instead of trying to overhaul your entire life at once, focus on small, achievable changes. This could be something like adding an extra serving of vegetables to your dinner or taking a 10-minute walk each day. Over time, these small changes can add up to big results.

Building healthy habits is another key strategy. Habits are actions that we do automatically, without having to think too much about them. By building healthy habits, you're making it easier to stick with your sustainable lifestyle over the long term. This could be anything from meal prepping on Sundays to ensure you have healthy meals ready for the week, to setting a regular bedtime to support quality sleep. Integrating self-care into your daily routine is also important. Self-care is all about taking time to nurture your physical, mental, and emotional well-being. This could be through a relaxing bath, a good book, or a hobby you love. Remember, self-care isn't selfish. It's a necessary part of maintaining a sustainable lifestyle.

Consistency and adaptability are crucial when it comes to maintaining a sustainable lifestyle. Consistency is about sticking with your healthy habits, even when life gets busy or challenging. It's about making your sustainable lifestyle a priority, no matter what else is going on. But life is unpredictable, and there will be times when sticking to your routine is difficult. That's where adaptability comes in. Adaptability is about being flexible and finding ways to maintain your sustainable lifestyle, even when things don't go as planned. This could mean having a backup plan for when you can't get to the gym, or finding healthy restaurant options when you're traveling. It's also important to have strategies for overcoming setbacks. Setbacks are a normal part of any journey, and they don't mean you've failed. Instead, they're an opportunity to learn and grow. When you encounter a setback, don't dwell on it. Instead, focus on what you can do differently next time. And remember, staying motivated is key. Find what inspires you, whether it's a supportive community, a personal goal, or simply the desire to feel your best.

Community and social support play a significant role in sustaining healthy lifestyle changes. Having a support system can make all the difference when it comes to sticking with your sustainable lifestyle. This could be family members who encourage your healthy eating habits, friends who join you for regular workouts, or online networks that provide motivation and advice. Don't underestimate the power of community. Sharing your journey with others can provide accountability, encouragement, and a sense of belonging. Plus, it's a great way to learn from others and gain new insights and strategies for maintaining your sustainable lifestyle. So, reach out, connect, and build your support network. It's an investment in your long-term success.

There are countless examples of sustainable lifestyle changes that support heart health. Meal prepping is a great one. By setting aside time each week to prepare healthy meals, you're setting yourself up for success. It makes it easier to stick with your healthy eating habits, even on busy days. Regular exercise is another example. This could be anything from a daily walk to a weekly yoga class. The key is to find something you enjoy and can stick with over the long term. Mindfulness practices, like meditation or deep breathing, are also powerful tools for supporting heart health. They help manage stress, which is a major risk factor for heart disease. Other examples include staying hydrated, getting quality sleep, and reducing your exposure to toxins. Remember, a sustainable lifestyle is all about finding what works for you. So, explore different options, and don't be afraid to think outside the box.

While creating a sustainable lifestyle is incredibly beneficial, it's not without its challenges. Common barriers include time constraints, lack of motivation, and environmental factors. But with a little creativity and determination, these barriers can be overcome. For time constraints, remember that even small changes can make a big difference. You don't need to spend hours at the gym or in the kitchen to support your heart health. Even a 10-minute walk or a quick, healthy meal can be beneficial. When it comes to motivation, find what inspires you. This could be a personal goal, a supportive community, or simply the desire to feel your best. And for environmental factors, do what you can to create a supportive environment.

This could mean stocking your kitchen with healthy foods, finding a workout buddy, or creating a relaxing bedtime routine. Remember, every challenge is an opportunity for growth. So, don't let barriers hold you back. Instead, find ways to work with them, and keep moving forward on your journey to a sustainable lifestyle.

The benefits of a sustainable lifestyle extend far beyond heart health. When you make choices that support your well-being, you're investing in your overall quality of life. This can mean improved energy, allowing you to tackle your day with vigor. It can mean mental clarity, helping you stay focused and productive. And it can mean resilience, giving you the strength to bounce back from life's challenges.

Plus, a sustainable lifestyle can support emotional well-being, providing a sense of balance and contentment. And let's not forget the physical benefits, from a strong, healthy body to a reduced risk of chronic disease. In short, a sustainable lifestyle is a gift you give yourself, a gift that keeps on giving, enhancing every aspect of your life.

Let's look at a case study to bring all these concepts to life. Meet John, a 45-year-old man who was diagnosed with high blood pressure. Determined to take control of his health, John decided to create a sustainable lifestyle that supports heart health. He started by setting realistic goals, like cooking at home more often and taking a daily walk. He built healthy habits, like meal prepping on Sundays and setting a regular bedtime. He found ways to integrate self-care into his routine, like reading before bed and joining a local hiking group. John also focused on consistency and adaptability. He stuck with his healthy habits, even when life got busy, and found ways to work around challenges, like bad weather or travel. He also leaned on his community for support, from his family who encouraged his healthy eating habits to his hiking group who kept him motivated. Over time, John's sustainable lifestyle paid off. His blood pressure improved, he had more energy, and he felt better overall. Plus, he found that his sustainable lifestyle had benefits beyond heart health. He was more productive at work, had better relationships, and felt a sense of accomplishment and contentment. John's story is a testament to the power of a sustainable lifestyle. It's a journey, one that requires commitment and determination, but the rewards are well worth the effort.

In conclusion, creating a sustainable lifestyle that supports heart health is a journey, one that requires commitment, determination, and a willingness to make changes. But it's a journey that's well worth the effort. By focusing on key components like nutrition, exercise, stress management, sleep, and toxin reduction, you're investing in your long-term well-being. By setting realistic goals, building healthy habits, and integrating self-care into your routine, you're setting yourself up for success. And by leaning on your community for support, you're making it easier to stick with your sustainable lifestyle over the long term. Remember, every choice you make is an opportunity to support your heart health and overall well-being. So, take it one step at a time, and don't be afraid to ask for help along the way. Your heart, and your overall health, will thank you.

Inspiring Stories of Individuals Who Reversed Heart Disease Naturally

There's a quiet revolution happening in heart health -- one that doesn't rely on prescription pads, surgical suites, or the cold authority of white coats. It's the story of real people who took back control of their bodies, defied the grim prognoses handed to them, and reversed heart disease using nothing more than the wisdom of nature, the power of food, and the resilience of the human spirit. These are not fairy tales or outliers; they are documented transformations that prove the body's astonishing capacity to heal when given the right tools. And here's the most empowering truth of all: if they can do it, so can you.

Take the story of Doug, a 58-year-old former construction worker from Texas who was told by his cardiologist that his arteries were so clogged he'd need a triple bypass within months -- or risk a fatal heart attack. The doctor's parting words? "There's nothing else you can do." But Doug wasn't ready to surrender. He dug into research outside the mainstream, discovering the work of doctors like Caldwell Esselstyn, who'd shown that a whole-food, plant-based diet could not only halt heart disease but reverse it. Within weeks, Doug overhauled his pantry, swapping processed meats and fried foods for leafy greens, berries, nuts, and legumes. He started walking daily, then jogging, and within six months, his follow-up angiogram stunned his cardiologist: his arteries had cleared significantly. No surgery. No stents. Just his body, healing itself. Doug's story isn't unique -- it's a blueprint. His success hinged on three things: refusing to accept "no" as the final answer, educating himself beyond the limits of conventional medicine, and surrounding himself with a community of others who'd done the same.

Then there's Maria, a 62-year-old schoolteacher from Florida whose high blood pressure and atrial fibrillation had her on a cocktail of five medications. She'd resigned herself to a life of side effects -- fatigue, dizziness, and a nagging fear that her heart would give out during class. But after attending a local workshop on natural heart health, she learned about the role of magnesium deficiency in arrhythmias and the inflammatory effects of processed foods. Maria began juicing organic vegetables, supplementing with magnesium and CoQ10, and practicing deep breathing exercises to manage stress. Within three months, her blood pressure normalized, and her cardiologist -- initially skeptical -- began tapering her off medications. The turning point? Maria realized her body wasn't broken; it was starving for the right nutrients and drowning in toxins. Her journey wasn't easy -- friends called her "obsessive," and her first attempt at a green juice ended in the sink -- but she persisted because she'd tasted what freedom from fear felt like.

What these stories share isn't just a happy ending; it's a set of principles that anyone can apply. First, education is power. Every person who reversed their heart disease became a student of their own body, questioning the status quo and seeking out alternative voices -- voices often silenced by an industry that profits from chronic illness. Second, support networks matter. Whether it was online forums, local meetups, or family members who joined them in the kitchen, none of these individuals did it alone. Third, personalization is key. There's no one-size-fits-all "heart healing" diet or protocol. Doug thrived on a plant-based approach, while Maria needed targeted supplements and stress reduction. The common thread? They listened to their bodies, not just their doctors.

Of course, the road wasn't smooth. Many faced resistance from conventional healthcare providers who dismissed their choices as "dangerous" or "unproven." Some were told they were "playing with fire" by stopping medications or refusing procedures. Others dealt with skepticism from loved ones who'd bought into the narrative that heart disease is a one-way street -- manageable only with drugs and surgeries. And let's not sugarcoat the setbacks: there were moments of doubt, cravings for old comfort foods, and days when progress felt invisible. But here's the thing about natural healing -- it's not a quick fix. It's a recommitment to life, one meal, one breath, one step at a time. The people who succeed are the ones who see those challenges not as failures, but as part of the process.

One of the most damaging myths about reversing heart disease naturally is that it's only possible for "mild" cases or requires extreme, unsustainable measures. Nothing could be further from the truth. The research -- much of it buried by institutions that stand to lose billions if people start healing themselves -- shows that even advanced atherosclerosis can be reversed with dietary and lifestyle changes. Dr. Dean Ornish's landmark studies proved this decades ago, yet how many cardiologists mention his work to their patients? The reality is, the body is designed to heal. Clogged arteries aren't a life sentence; they're a wake-up call. And the "extreme" measures? They're only extreme compared to a culture that sees popping a pill as easier than eating a vegetable. But when you've stared down the barrel of a heart attack, "extreme" starts to look a lot like common sense.

Hope is the fuel that keeps people going when the path gets tough. It's what gets someone like James, a 45-year-old father of two, to swap his fast-food habit for home-cooked meals after a scare with chest pains. It's what pushes Linda, a retired nurse, to start a garden so she can grow her own organic produce after decades of trusting the system that failed her. Hope isn't naive; it's radical. It's the belief that your body is not a ticking time bomb but a self-repairing masterpiece, waiting for the right conditions to thrive. And here's the beautiful part: hope is contagious. When you hear these stories, something shifts. The "what if" becomes "why not me?"

Community plays a role that can't be overstated. In a world where Big Pharma's ads dominate the airwaves and doctors' visits are rushed and impersonal, finding a tribe of like-minded people can mean the difference between giving up and pushing through. Online groups, local co-ops, and even simple accountability partners provide the encouragement and practical tips that make the journey feel less lonely. They're the ones who'll share their favorite kale recipe, remind you to take your deep breaths when stress hits, or celebrate with you when your cholesterol numbers drop. Healing isn't just a physical process; it's a social one. We're wired to thrive in connection, not isolation.

So where do you start? Right where you are. Maybe it's swapping your morning cereal for a smoothie packed with spinach, blueberries, and flaxseeds. Maybe it's a 10-minute walk after dinner, or five minutes of quiet breathing before bed. Maybe it's just the decision to question the next prescription you're handed and ask, "Is there another way?" The people in these stories didn't have superhuman willpower or secret knowledge. They had something far more powerful: the courage to take the first step. And then the next. That's how transformations begin -- not with a grand gesture, but with a single choice to trust yourself more than the system.

The system, after all, wasn't built to heal you. It was built to manage you -- to keep you dependent on pills, procedures, and the illusion that you're powerless without them. But you're not powerless. Your heart doesn't belong to a pharmaceutical company or a hospital board. It belongs to you. And it's waiting for you to reclaim it. These stories aren't just inspiration; they're proof. Proof that the body can heal, that nature provides the medicine, and that the greatest authority on your health isn't someone in a white coat -- it's you.

Integrative Cardiology: IV Therapies, Antioxidants, Platelet Infusions, Ozone, Exosomes, Stem cell Therapy

Imagine for a moment that your heart isn't just a pump, but a finely tuned engine -- one that thrives not just on fuel, but on the right kind of care. Now, what if the best way to keep that engine running smoothly wasn't just popping a pill prescribed by a system that profits from your sickness? What if the real answers lay in therapies that work with your body's natural healing abilities, not against them? That's the promise of integrative cardiology -- a field that refuses to be boxed in by the dogma of Big Pharma or the limitations of a broken medical system.

Integrative cardiology is about reclaiming control over your heart health by blending the best of time-tested natural therapies with the precision of modern science -- without the toxic side effects of synthetic drugs. It's a rebellion against the idea that heart disease is an inevitable sentence, handed down by a system that would rather manage your decline than empower your recovery. At its core, integrative cardiology recognizes that your heart doesn't exist in isolation. It's deeply connected to your diet, your stress levels, your gut health, and even the quality of the air you breathe. So instead of treating symptoms with a one-size-fits-all drug, it focuses on therapies that address the root causes of cardiovascular decline: chronic inflammation, poor circulation, cellular damage, and nutritional deficiencies.

What is the NLRP3 Inflammasome?

Imagine your body as a fortress, constantly under siege by invisible invaders --toxins from processed foods, stress hormones from a chaotic world, and metabolic chaos from poor sleep or sugar binges. Inside this fortress, you've got a highly trained security team ready to sound the alarm at the first sign of trouble. That team is your immune system, and one of its most powerful tools is something called the NLRP3 inflammasome. You've probably never heard of it, but if you care about your heart, your brain, or even your energy levels, this tiny molecular machine could be the difference between vibrant health and chronic disease.

So, what exactly is the NLRP3 inflammasome? Think of it as a cellular fire alarm. It's a multi-protein complex inside your immune cells that acts like a sensor for danger. When it detects threats -- like bacterial toxins, excessive oxidative stress, or even tiny crystals from damaged cells -- it springs into action. The NLRP3 inflammasome assembles like a puzzle, triggering a cascade that releases inflammatory signals, most notably a molecule called interleukin-1 beta (IL-1β). This is your body's way of saying, "Hey, we've got a problem here!" In short bursts, this inflammation is protective. It helps isolate infections, clear out debris, and jumpstart repairs. But when the NLRP3 inflammasome gets stuck in the "on" position -- thanks to chronic stress, poor diet, or environmental toxins -- it becomes like a fire alarm that won't stop blaring. The result? A slow, smoldering inflammation that damages your arteries, weakens your heart, and accelerates aging.

Now, here's where things get personal for your heart. The NLRP3 inflammasome doesn't just respond to infections -- it's hyper-sensitive to the modern lifestyle.

Processed foods loaded with seed oils, high-fructose corn syrup, and artificial additives? They're like fuel on the fire, activating NLRP3 and driving up inflammation. Chronic stress from financial worries, relationship struggles, or even the nonstop news cycle? That cranks up cortisol, which in turn revs up NLRP3. Even seemingly harmless habits, like sitting too much or skimping on sleep, can trigger this inflammasome, setting off a chain reaction that harms your endothelial cells -- the delicate lining of your blood vessels. Over time, this leads to stiffness in your arteries, plaque buildup, and the kind of silent inflammation that paves the way for heart attacks and strokes.

But the NLRP3 inflammasome's role in heart disease goes deeper than just inflammation. Research has shown it's a key player in atherosclerosis, the process where your arteries clog up like a drain full of grease. When LDL cholesterol (the so-called "bad" cholesterol, though the real villain is oxidized LDL seeps into your artery walls, your immune cells rush in to clean up the mess. But if NLRP3 is overactive, those immune cells go rogue, releasing too much IL-1β and turning the artery wall into a battleground. The result? Plaques grow larger, become unstable, and eventually rupture -- triggering a heart attack. NLRP3 also worsens hypertension by promoting stiffness in your blood vessels and disrupting the balance of salts and fluids in your body. And if you've ever heard of heart failure, where the heart gradually weakens and can't pump effectively, NLRP3 is often pulling the strings there too, driving the fibrosis (scarring that turns a strong heart muscle into a flabby, inefficient one.

You might be thinking, "Okay, so NLRP3 is bad news. What can I actually do about it?" Here's the good news: unlike some genetic time bombs, the NLRP3 inflammasome is highly responsive to your lifestyle. That means you've got leverage. Start with your plate. Foods rich in polyphenols -- think berries, dark leafy greens, turmeric, and green tea -- act like natural NLRP3 inhibitors. These compounds calm the inflammasome by neutralizing oxidative stress and reducing the signals that trigger its activation. On the flip side, cut out the inflammasome's favorite fuels: refined sugars, trans fats, and processed meats. These aren't just empty calories; they're direct activators of NLRP3, turning every meal into a silent inflammatory assault.

Then there's stress -- a major, often overlooked NLRP3 trigger. When you're stuck in fight-or-flight mode, your body pumps out stress hormones that prime the inflammasome for overreaction. This is why practices like deep breathing, forest bathing (yes, just being in nature), and even laughter aren't just "woo-woo" advice. They literally dial down NLRP3 activity by lowering cortisol and boosting your body's natural anti-inflammatory defenses. Sleep is another non-negotiable. Poor sleep doesn't just leave you groggy; it spikes inflammatory markers, including IL-1β, and makes your NLRP3 inflammasome hypersensitive. Aim for 7-9 hours in a dark, cool room -- your heart will thank you.

Detoxification is another critical but often ignored strategy. Your body is constantly bombarded with NLRP3 activators -- heavy metals like mercury from dental fillings or fish, glyphosate from non-organic foods, and even microplastics lurking in your water. These toxins accumulate in your tissues, keeping the inflammasome on high alert. Supporting your liver with milk thistle, sweating out toxins in a sauna, and drinking clean, filtered water can help reduce this burden. And don't underestimate the power of movement. Exercise, especially strength training and high-intensity intervals, helps regulate NLRP3 by improving insulin sensitivity, reducing visceral fat (a major inflammasome activator), and boosting your body's antioxidant defenses.

If you're dealing with existing heart issues or want an extra layer of protection, targeted supplements can be game-changers. Magnesium, for instance, is a natural NLRP3 inhibitor -- it helps stabilize the inflammasome and reduces IL-1β production. Vitamin D, often deficient in those with chronic inflammation, also modulates NLRP3 activity. Then there's sulforaphane, a compound found in broccoli sprouts, which has been shown in studies to directly inhibit NLRP3 activation. Even spices like ginger and garlic aren't just flavor enhancers; they contain bioactive compounds that help keep this inflammasome in check. For those who need more support, herbs like berberine and resveratrol have been studied for their ability to down-regulate NLRP3, offering a natural alternative to pharmaceuticals that come with a laundry list of side effects.

Let's bust a couple of myths while we're at it. First, the idea that NLRP3 is only relevant if you have an autoimmune disease is flat-out wrong. This inflammasome is a universal player in chronic disease, from heart disease to diabetes to Alzheimer's. If you've got inflammation, NLRP3 is almost certainly involved.

Second, the notion that you can't influence NLRP3 with lifestyle is a dangerous lie perpetuated by a medical system that would rather prescribe a pill than empower you to take control. The truth? Your daily choices -- what you eat, how you move, how you manage stress and the integrative therapies described later in this chapter-- are the most powerful tools you have to modulate this inflammasome.

Big Pharma would love for you to believe otherwise and is already actively studying monoclonal antibodies that will look to impact your NLRP3 Inflammasome recognizing how the cholesterol hypothesis has failed them with regard to reducing cardiovascular events.

When I spoke to the lead investigator from Harvard about these studies he answered with excitement with regard to these monoclonal antibodies and felt that these natural and further intravenous techniques that will be described later in this chapter are not as effective. When asked further, he denied ever looking into these modalities but was excited to promote the Big Pharma sponsor of these monoclonal antibodies. I think it escapes no one's attention that he makes money by running these studies. He admitted he never looked into them deeply enough.

Take the case of Mark, a 58-year-old man who came to me with high blood pressure, borderline diabetes, and a family history of heart disease. His doctor had him on three medications, with a fourth on the horizon. Mark was skeptical when I told him his issues might be driven by an overactive NLRP3 inflammasome, but he was willing to try a natural approach. We started by cleaning up his diet --out went the processed foods, in came wild-caught fish, organic veggies, and berries. He began walking daily and added a 10-minute meditation to his mornings. Within weeks, his blood pressure started dropping. Three months later, he'd lost 15 pounds, his fasting blood sugar was normal, and his doctor took him off one of his medications. A year in, Mark's inflammatory markers had plummeted, and his arteries showed less stiffness on tests. His story isn't unique --it's what happens when you address the root cause (in his case, a hyperactive NLRP3 instead of just slapping a Band-Aid on symptoms.)

The bottom line? The NLRP3 inflammasome isn't some obscure scientific curiosity -- it's a central player in your heart health, and you've got more control over it than you realize. The same system that's designed to protect you can turn against you when bombarded by modern life's toxic cocktail. But here's the empowering part: every bite of real food, every deep breath, every night of restorative sleep, and every detoxifying sweat session, and the integrative therapies described below, is a vote for a calmer, more balanced inflammasome. You don't need to wait for some pharmaceutical breakthrough or government health guidelines to take action. The tools are already in your hands --literally. Your heart's future isn't written in stone; it's written in the choices you make today. And those choices can either fan the flames of inflammation or extinguish them for good.

Intravenous (IV) Therapies:

Let's start with one of the most powerful tools in this arsenal: Intravenous (IV) nutrient and anti-inflammatory therapies. This isn't your average vitamin supplement. It's a targeted, high-dose infusion of essential nutrients like vitamin C, magnesium, and B vitamins -- delivered straight into your bloodstream where they can bypass a sluggish digestive system and get to work immediately. Studies have shown that **IV vitamin C**, for example, can dramatically reduce inflammation in the arteries, a key driver of atherosclerosis. **Magnesium**, often called the 'relaxation mineral,' helps regulate blood pressure and prevent dangerous arrhythmias. And B vitamins?

They're critical for homocysteine metabolism -- a marker that, when elevated, is a stronger predictor of heart disease than cholesterol ever was. They also are essential in optimizining mitochondrial function.

IV Phosphatidylcholine/Plaquex Therapy: Structure and Function

Phosphatidylcholine is a phospholipid, a major component of cell membranes, and a crucial factor in maintaining cellular structure and function (Gatt, 2021). It plays vital roles in lipid metabolism, membrane fluidity, and signal transduction.

Mechanisms of Action

Plaque Regression: IV Plaquex target and regress atherosclerotic plaques by:

Emulsifying and Dissolving Plaque: Plaquex forms micelles that encapsulate and dissolve cholesterol crystals, promoting plaque regression (Gatt, 2021).

Inhibiting Foam Cell Formation: Plaquex inhibits the transformation of macrophages into foam cells, preventing further plaque growth (Gatt, 2021).

Improving Lipid Profile: IV Plaquex can improve lipid profiles by:

Reducing Total Cholesterol and LDL-C: Plaquex reduces total cholesterol and LDL-C levels by promoting cholesterol efflux from macrophages and enhancing hepatic cholesterol clearance (Gatt, 2021).

Increasing HDL-C: Plaquex increases HDL-C levels, which facilitates reverse cholesterol transport (Gatt, 2021).

Enhancing Endothelial Function: IV Plaquex can improve endothelial function by:

Stimulating Nitric Oxide (NO) Production: PC activates endothelial nitric oxide synthase (eNOS), increasing NO production and enhancing endothelial function (Gatt, 2021).

Reducing Inflammation: PC reduces inflammation by modulating immune cell function and decreasing pro-inflammatory cytokine release (Gatt, 2021).

Reducing Oxidative Stress: IV PC and IV Plaquex can decrease oxidative stress by

Scavenging Reactive Oxygen Species (ROS): Plaquex acts as an antioxidant, neutralizing ROS and preventing oxidative damage (Gatt, 2021).

Enhancing Antioxidant Enzyme Activity: Plaquex increases the activity of antioxidant enzymes, such as superoxide dismutase (SOD) and catalase (Gatt, 2021).

Plaquex have been used clinically for over three decades, demonstrating safety and efficacy in numerous studies (Gatt, 2021). Commonly reported side effects are minor and include flushing, nausea, and temporary discomfort at the injection site. Contraindications include severe hypersensitivity to PC, pregnancy, and breastfeeding.

IV Curcumin

Curcumin is a potent bioactive compound derived from turmeric, has garnered significant attention in treating cardiovascular disease (CVD).

Mechanisms of Action

IV curcumin exerts its cardioprotective effects through various mechanisms:

Anti-inflammatory and Anti-oxidant Effects: Curcumin reduces oxidative stress and inflammation by scavenging reactive oxygen species (ROS) and inhibiting the production of pro-inflammatory cytokines (Panahi et al., 2018).

Anti-thrombotic and Anti-aggregatory Effects: Curcumin inhibits platelet aggregation and thrombus formation, reducing the risk of CVD events (Panahi et al., 2018).

Vasodilatory Effects: Curcumin induces vasodilation by activating potassium channels and inhibiting calcium influx, improving blood flow and reducing afterload (Panahi et al., 2018).

Anti-apoptotic Effects: Curcumin protects cardiomyocytes from apoptosis by activating the PI3K/Akt signaling pathway (Panahi et al., 2018).

Modulation of Lipid Profile: Curcumin reduces total cholesterol, LDL-C, and triglycerides, while increasing HDL-C levels (Panahi et al., 2018).

Clinical Applications

Acute Coronary Syndromes: IV curcumin has been used in the management of acute coronary syndromes, reducing chest pain, improving myocardial perfusion, and decreasing infarct size (Panahi et al., 2018).

Heart Failure: Curcumin has shown potential in treating heart failure by improving cardiac function, reducing inflammation, and enhancing quality of life (Panahi et al., 2018).

Peripheral Artery Disease: IV curcumin can improve walking distance and reduce symptoms in patients with peripheral artery disease (Panahi et al., 2018).

IV Curcumin is generally safe and well-tolerated. Minor side effects, such as temporary numbness, tingling, or metallic taste, may occur. Contraindications include hypersensitivity to curcumin, severe heart block, and severe hypotension (Panahi et al., 2018).

IV Epigallocatechin Gallate (EGCG)

EGCG is, a potent polyphenol found in green tea, which has demonstrated significant impact in treating cardiovascular disease (CVD).

Mechanisms of Action

IV EGCG exerts its cardioprotective effects through various mechanisms:

Anti-inflammatory and Anti-oxidant Effects: EGCG reduces oxidative stress and inflammation by scavenging reactive oxygen species (ROS) and inhibiting the production of pro-inflammatory cytokines (Khan & Mukhtar, 2018).

Anti-thrombotic and Anti-aggregatory Effects: EGCG inhibits platelet aggregation and thrombus formation, reducing the risk of CVD events (Khan & Mukhtar, 2018).

Vasodilatory Effects: EGCG induces vasodilation by activating potassium channels and inhibiting calcium influx, improving blood flow and reducing afterload (Khan & Mukhtar, 2018).

Anti-apoptotic Effects: EGCG protects cardiomyocytes from apoptosis by activating the PI3K/Akt signaling pathway (Khan & Mukhtar, 2018).

Modulation of Lipid Profile: EGCG reduces total cholesterol, LDL-C, and triglycerides, while increasing HDL-C levels (Khan & Mukhtar, 2018).

Inhibition of Atherosclerosis: EGCG inhibits atherosclerosis by preventing foam cell formation and stabilizing atherosclerotic plaques (Khan & Mukhtar, 2018).

IV Taurine administration has garnered interest in cardiovascular disease management due to its potential benefits. Taurine, a sulfur-containing amino acid, is abundant in food products and is generally recognized as safe and has been shown to exert cardioprotective effects by modulating various pathways. It scavenges reactive oxygen species, stabilizes membranes, and regulates intracellular calcium homeostasis (Huxtable, 1992). It improves cardiac function in various cardiovascular diseases. A study in patients with chronic heart failure demonstrated that iv taurine infusion improved left ventricular ejection fraction and reduced brain natriuretic peptide levels (Matsumoto et al., 2006).

Reduced Inflammation and Oxidative Stress: Taurine has anti-inflammatory and antioxidant properties creating a Teflon like charge to endothelial lining making it resistant to oxidized LDL. (Schaffer et al., 2000) (Cholesterol Sulfate deficiency causes atherosclerosis, Seneff et al., 2018).

Anti-Arrhythmic Effects: Iv taurine has shown potential anti-arrhythmic effects in animal models. It may help prevent or treat arrhythmias associated with cardiovascular diseases (Li et al., 2014).

Then there's the game-changing role of antioxidants -- not just in pill form, but delivered intravenously or through foods like cocoa and beetroot, which are packed with flavonoids that actively reverse vascular damage. Research published on NaturalNews.com in 2025 revealed that flavanol-rich cocoa can neutralize the arterial stiffness caused by prolonged sitting -- something that plagues millions in our sedentary, screen-bound culture. Beetroot juice, meanwhile, is a nitric oxide powerhouse, dilating blood vessels to improve circulation and lower blood pressure naturally. These aren't fringe ideas; they're backed by science that Big Pharma would rather you ignore because they can't patent a beet. The supplement industry has now developed multiple compounds that are all natural and not only boost nitric oxide levels but destroy the concomitant peroxynitrates that are formed boosting the longevity of nitric oxide.

Now, let's talk about therapies that sound like they're straight out of a sci-fi novel but are very real and increasingly accessible: platelet-rich plasma/fibrinogen (PRP therapy), ozone therapy, exosome therapy, and stem cell treatments.

PRP/F involves drawing a small amount of your own blood, concentrating the platelets (which are packed with growth factors, and reinjecting them into damaged heart tissue. The infusions promote healing and tissue repair through the wealth of healing factors that platelets are designed to carry to every part of your body.

Platelets and Growth Factors: PRP is rich in platelets, which contain numerous growth factors essential for tissue healing and regeneration. These growth factors include:

Platelet-Derived Growth Factor (PDGF): Promotes cell growth and division, particularly fibroblasts and smooth muscle cells.

Transforming Growth Factor-β (TGF-β): Regulates cell growth, cell differentiation, and cell proliferation.

Vascular Endothelial Growth Factor (VEGF): Stimulates angiogenesis, the formation of new blood vessels.

Fibroblast Growth Factor (FGF): Promotes cell growth and division, particularly fibroblasts.

Epidermal Growth Factor (EGF): Stimulates cell growth and differentiation, particularly in epithelial cells.

Insulin-like Growth Factor (IGF): Promotes cell growth and division.

Cytokines: PRP contains various cytokines that play crucial roles in inflammation modulation, cell signaling, and immune response. Some key cytokines in PRP include:

Interleukin-1β (IL-1β): Regulates the inflammatory response and stimulates the production of other cytokines.

Interleukin-8 (IL-8): A potent chemoattractant for neutrophils and promotes angiogenesis.

Interleukin-10 (IL-10): Has anti-inflammatory properties and regulates the immune response.

Fibrinogen and Fibrin: PRP contains fibrinogen, which, upon activation, forms a fibrin network that result in accelerated healing and reduced scar tissue in hearts weakened by heart attacks or chronic ischemia.

Ozone therapy, often dismissed by mainstream medicine as 'quackery,' can be given via the oral, rectal, dermal and most powerfully via IV Infusions (never by direct IV infusion of the gas known as "DIV").

It works by introducing medical-grade ozone into the bloodstream, which stimulates the production of hermetic ROS, Ozonides and improves oxygen utilization by mitochondria, and even helps break down arterial plaque.

Ozone Therapy: Mechanisms of Action

Ozone therapy increases oxygen utilization by red blood cells, enhancing oxygen delivery to tissues and improving mitochondrial function (Viebahn-Haensler, 2003).

Increased Antioxidant Enzymes: Ozone stimulates the production of antioxidant enzymes, such as superoxide dismutase (SOD), catalase, and glutathione peroxidase, which protect cells from oxidative damage (Viebahn-Haensler, 2003).

Regulation of Inflammation: Ozone therapy modulates the inflammatory response by activating immune cells and promoting the release of anti-inflammatory cytokines (Viebahn-Haensler, 2003).

Improved Endothelial Function: Ozone enhances endothelial nitric oxide synthase (eNOS) activity, leading to increased nitric oxide (NO) production and improved endothelial function (Viebahn-Haensler, 2003).

Ozone Therapy via EBOO and MAH for CVD

EBOO: In EBOO, Large volumes of blood (anywhere between 2-4 Liters) is withdrawn from the patient, exposed to ozone, and then immediately reinfused. The protocol can vary and in general more ozonides are produced (80%) vs ROS (20%) This method allows for precise control of ozone dosage and minimizes side effects (Viebahn-Haensler, 2003).

MAH: In MAH, a small volume of blood is withdrawn, ozonated, and then reinjected intramuscularly. Larger amounts can be infused via IV (usually 250cc-2 Liters) MAH is simpler to administer but offers less precise control over ozone dosage and creates more ROS (80%) than Ozonides (20%) (Viebahn-Haensler, 2003).

Benefits for CVD

Reversal of Atherosclerosis: Ozone therapy has been shown to reverse atherosclerosis by promoting cholesterol efflux, reducing oxidative stress, and modulating inflammation (Viebahn-Haensler, 2003).

Improved Angina Symptoms: Ozone therapy has been found to alleviate angina symptoms by enhancing myocardial oxygen supply and improving endothelial function (Viebahn-Haensler, 2003).

Reduced Ischemia-Reperfusion Injury: Ozone pre-conditioning has been demonstrated to protect against ischemia-reperfusion injury, reducing myocardial damage and improving cardiac function (Viebahn-Haensler, 2003).

Safety and Contraindications

Ozone therapy is generally safe and well-tolerated. Contraindications include severe anemia, pregnancy, and certain blood disorders (Viebahn-Haensler, 2003).

Exosomes

Exosomes act like molecular messengers, signaling damaged heart cells to regenerate. These are nanovesicles that can be released by various cell types, but the primary focus here is on umbilical cord and placental mesenchymal cells, and autologous stem cells.

These have emerged as therapeutic agents for treating cardiovascular diseases (CVD).

Exosomes are 40-160 nm vesicles derived from the endosomal compartment, containing proteins, lipids, and nucleic acids (RNA and DNA) that reflect the parental cell's phenotype (Tkach & Thery, 2016). Most importantly this is an acellular process. This is important to note for those concerned about receiving foreign cells in their body. They mediate cell-to-cell communication by transferring their cargo to recipient cells, modulating their function and phenotype. Exosomes can be separate and categorized to treat specific ailments.

Exosomes in Cardiovascular Disease

1. ***Angiogenesis and Vasculogenesis:*** Exosomes derived from various cell types, such as endothelial progenitor cells (EPCs) and mesenchymal stem cells (MSCs), promote angiogenesis and vasculogenesis by carrying pro-angiogenic factors like VEGF, FGF, and SDF-1 (Tkach & Thery, 2016).

2. ***Anti-inflammatory and Anti-fibrotic Effects:*** Exosomes can modulate the immune response and reduce inflammation, thereby attenuating CVD progression. For instance, MSC-derived exosomes can decrease macrophage infiltration and reduce fibrosis in myocardial infarction (MI) models (Tkach & Thery, 2016).

3. ***Regeneration and Repair:*** Exosomes can stimulate the proliferation and differentiation of resident cardiac stem cells, promoting heart regeneration and repair following injury (Tkach & Thery, 2016).

4. ***Cholesterol Efflux:*** Exosomes can facilitate cholesterol efflux from macrophages, reducing foam cell formation and atherosclerosis progression (Tkach & Thery, 2016).

Clinical Applications of Exosomes in CVD

1. ***Ischemic Heart Disease:*** Exosome therapy has shown promise in treating ischemic heart disease, improving cardiac function, and reducing infarct size in preclinical models (Tkach & Thery, 2016).

2. ***Atherosclerosis:*** Exosomes can modulate immune responses and promote cholesterol efflux, making them potential therapeutics for atherosclerosis (Tkach & Thery, 2016).

3. ***Heart Failure:*** Exosome-based therapies have demonstrated potential in treating heart failure by promoting cardiac regeneration, reducing fibrosis, and improving cardiac function (Tkach & Thery, 2016).

Safety and Challenges

Exosomes are generally considered safe, however, challenges remain regarding their large-scale production, standardization, and long-term safety (Tkach & Thery, 2016). Additionally, the optimal exosome source, dose, and delivery method require further investigation.

Stem Cell Infusions

Stem Cells have emerged as a powerful natural and regenerative approach to treating cardiovascular disease (CVD). This essay explores the mechanisms, clinical applications, safety, and efficacy of stem cell infusions in CVD treatment.

Mechanisms of Action

Stem cell infusions exert their cardioprotective effects through various mechanisms:

Regenerative Potential: Stem cells differentiate into functional cardiomyocytes, vascular endothelial cells, and smooth muscle cells, replacing damaged tissue and restoring normal cardiac function (Makkar et al., 2012).

Paracrine Effects: Stem cells secrete growth factors, cytokines, and exosomes that promote angiogenesis, reduce inflammation, and inhibit apoptosis (Makkar et al., 2012).

Modulation of Immune Response: Stem cells modulate the immune response by promoting regulatory T cells and inhibiting pro-inflammatory cytokines (Makkar et al., 2012).

Improvement of Microvascular Function: Stem cells enhance microvascular function and perfusion, reducing ischemia and promoting tissue repair (Makkar et al., 2012).

Clinical Applications

Ischemic Heart Disease: Stem cell infusions have demonstrated benefits in treating ischemic heart disease by improving left ventricular ejection fraction, reducing infarct size, and enhancing quality of life (Makkar et al., 2012).

Heart Failure: Stem cell therapy has demonstrated potential in treating heart failure by improving cardiac function, reducing hospitalization, and enhancing survival (Makkar et al., 2012).

Peripheral Artery Disease: Stem cell infusions can improve walking distance and reduce symptoms in patients with peripheral artery disease (Makkar et al., 2012).

Safety and Efficacy

Stem cell infusions are generally safe and well-tolerated. They require close monitoring during infusion to assess if antihistamines or corticosteroids are warranted. These agents may also need to proceed infusion depending on previous reactions or dose. Minor side effects, such as temporary numbness, tingling, or metallic taste, may occur. Contraindications include hypersensitivity to stem cells, severe heart block, and severe hypotension (Makkar et al., 2012). Clinical studies have demonstrated the safety and efficacy of stem cell infusions in CVD treatment (Makkar et al., 2012)

IV Chelation Therapy

A process that removes heavy metals and other toxins from the body, has demonstrated significant benefits in treating cardiovascular disease (CVD).

Mechanisms of Action

IV chelation therapy exerts its cardioprotective effects through various mechanisms:

Heavy Metal Detoxification: Chelators such as ethylenediaminetetraacetic acid (EDTA) bind to heavy metals like lead, cadmium, and mercury, facilitating their elimination from the body (Eliaz et al., 2000).

Anti-inflammatory and Anti-oxidant Effects: Chelation reduces oxidative stress and inflammation by scavenging reactive oxygen species (ROS) and inhibiting the production of pro-inflammatory cytokines (Eliaz et al., 2000).

Improvement of Endothelial Function: Chelation enhances endothelial function by increasing nitric oxide (NO) bioavailability and reducing inflammation (Eliaz et al., 2000).

Modulation of Lipid Profile: Chelation reduces total cholesterol, LDL-C, and triglycerides, while increasing HDL-C levels (Eliaz et al., 2000).

Inhibition of Atherosclerosis: Chelation inhibits atherosclerosis by preventing foam cell formation and stabilizing atherosclerotic plaques (Eliaz et al., 2000).

Clinical Applications

Coronary Artery Disease: IV chelation therapy has shown promise in treating coronary artery disease by improving angina symptoms, enhancing myocardial perfusion, and reducing the need for revascularization procedures (Eliaz et al., 2000).

Peripheral Artery Disease: Chelation can improve walking distance and reduce symptoms in patients with peripheral artery disease (Eliaz et al., 2000).

Heart Failure: IV chelation therapy has demonstrated potential in treating heart failure by improving cardiac function, reducing hospitalization, and enhancing survival (Eliaz et al., 2000).

Safety and Efficacy

IV chelation therapy is generally safe and well-tolerated. Minor side effects, such as temporary numbness, tingling, or metallic taste, may occur. Contraindications include hypersensitivity to chelating agents, severe kidney disease, and severe hypotension (Eliaz et al., 2000). Clinical studies have demonstrated the safety and efficacy of IV chelation therapy in CVD treatment (Eliaz et al., 2000). The most prohibitive factor of IV chelation therapy is the attention involved during the procedure, the length of the IV infusions, and the need for monitoring for IV vitamin and mineral supplementation.

Plasmapheresis

A therapeutic apheresis technique involving the removal and separation of plasma from whole blood, through a few mechanisms.

Mechanical Separation: The core principle of apheresis is the mechanical separation of blood components based on their physical properties, such as size, density, and buoyancy. This is achieved using filtration techniques (Sethi et al., 2018). Plasma is separated from cellular components (red blood cells, white blood cells, and platelets) based on their density differences.

Adsorptive Processes: Some apheresis techniques, such as lipid apheresis and certain forms of plasmapheresis, employ adsorptive columns containing specific ligands or resins that bind to and remove targeted substances, such as lipoproteins or autoantibodies (Sethi et al., 2018). These adsorptive processes rely on chemical interactions rather than electrical charges.

Electrical Charges: Although electrical charges are not the primary mechanism, they do play a role in apheresis in the following ways:

Electrophoresis: In some apheresis techniques, an electric field is applied to separate charged molecules or particles based on their electrophoretic mobility. However, this is not the primary mechanism in most apheresis procedures (Sethi et al., 2018).

Plasmapheresis exerts its cardioprotective effects through various mechanisms:

Removal of Pathogenic Substances: Plasmapheresis removes harmful substances such as autoantibodies, immune complexes, and cytokines that contribute to CVD pathogenesis (Sethi et al., 2018).

Replacement with Fresh Frozen Plasma (FFP): The replacement of removed plasma with FFP replenishes essential clotting factors, proteins, and other plasma constituents, maintaining hemostasis (Sethi et al., 2018).

Modulation of Immune Response: Plasmapheresis modulates the immune response by reducing inflammation and inhibiting autoantibody production (Sethi et al., 2018).

Improvement of Microvascular Function: Plasmapheresis enhances microvascular function and perfusion, reducing ischemia and promoting tissue repair (Sethi et al., 2018).

Clinical Applications

Anti-phospholipid Syndrome (APS): Plasmapheresis is used in the management of APS, a CVD risk factor characterized by the presence of autoantibodies against phospholipids and coagulation proteins (Sethi et al., 2018).

Thrombotic Thrombocytopenic Purpura (TTP): Plasmapheresis is the first-line treatment for TTP, a life-threatening disorder characterized by thrombocytopenia, microangiopathic hemolytic anemia, and organ ischemia (Sethi et al., 2018).

Goodpasture Syndrome: Plasmapheresis is used in the treatment of Goodpasture syndrome, a rare autoimmune disorder characterized by glomerulonephritis and pulmonary hemorrhage (Sethi et al., 2018).

Cryoglobulinemia: Plasmapheresis is employed in the management of cryoglobulinemia, a disorder characterized by the presence of cryoglobulins, which can cause CVD manifestations (Sethi et al., 2018).

Dyslipidemia: Plasmapheresis has been used to treat adverse lipid panels where there are significantly elevated LP(a)'s which are genetic conditions that cannot be fully treated with medications or supplements and poses an increased cardiovascular risk to patients. In patients where there are also significant inflammatory components to their disease as measured by the blood work it can be very helpful in reducing the cytokine stimulation and inflammation that plays intricate role in coronary artery disease.

Safety and Efficacy

Plasmapheresis is generally safe and well-tolerated. Minor side effects, such as citrate reactions, hypocalcemia, and hypothermia, may occur. Contraindications include severe hypotension, hypovolemia, and active bleeding (Sethi et al., 2018).

Of course, the skeptics will say, 'But where's the proof?' The truth is, the proof is out there -- if you know where to look. Mainstream journals often ignore or suppress studies that don't align with the pharmaceutical narrative, but independent research and clinical experience tell a different story. For example, Dr. Caldwell Esselstyn's work on reversing heart disease through nutrition is well-documented, proving that even severe coronary artery disease can be halted and reversed with the right approach. Meanwhile, integrative cardiologists like Dr.

Sherry Rogers, have exposed the 'high blood pressure hoax,' showing how hypertension is often a symptom of deeper issues like magnesium deficiency or toxic exposure -- not a standalone condition requiring lifelong medication. The key is working with a provider who understands these therapies and knows how to tailor them to your unique biology.

One of the biggest myths about integrative cardiology is that it's only for the wealthy or the desperate. In reality, many of these therapies are more affordable than a lifetime of pharmaceuticals -- and far less costly than a heart attack or bypass surgery. IV therapies, for instance, can range from $100 to $300 per session, but when you compare that to the $30,000 price tag of a stent procedure (which often fails to address the root cause), the math starts to look very different. Stem cell therapy might seem expensive upfront, but for someone facing a heart transplant, it's a fraction of the cost -- and without the lifelong immunosuppressants. The real barrier isn't money; it's access to information.

Most people don't even know these options exist because their doctors are trained to push statins and blood pressure meds, not to explore alternatives that could actually heal.

Take the case of Mark, a 58-year-old man who came to an integrative cardiologist after suffering his second heart attack. His conventional doctors had him on five different medications, yet his ejection fraction -- a measure of how well his heart pumps -- was still dangerously low at 30%. Within six months of combining PRP therapy, ozone treatments, and a targeted nutrient protocol (including high-dose CoQ10 and magnesium, his ejection fraction improved to 55%. He was able to stop three of his medications entirely. Stories like Mark's aren't anomalies; they're what happens when you stop treating the heart as an isolated machine and start supporting the body's innate ability to heal.

So how do you access these therapies? Start by seeking out integrative cardiologists or functional medicine doctors who specialize in cardiovascular health. Look for providers who are transparent about their methods, willing to discuss risks and benefits openly, and who don't dismiss natural therapies as 'unproven' without having actually reviewed the evidence. Be wary of clinics that promise miracles -- real healing takes time and commitment -- but also don't let fearmongering from conventional doctors deter you. Remember, the same system that calls these therapies 'unproven' is the one that pushed statins on millions despite their well-documented muscle-destroying side effects, neurological disorders, liver inflammation and negligible impact on overall mortality.

References:

-Rogers, Sherry A. The High Blood Pressure Hoax

- *NaturalNews.com. Flavanol-Rich Foods Like Cocoa Can Neutralize Vascular Damage Caused by Prolonged Sitting. Lance D Johnson*
- *Esselstyn Jr, Caldwell B. Prevent and Reverse Heart Disease: The Revolutionary, Scientifically Proven, Nutrition-Based Cure*
- *NaturalNews.com. Curing Heart Disease: Practical Medical Solutions*
- *Mercola.com. Beetroot Juice Can Benefit Your Muscles*

About the Author

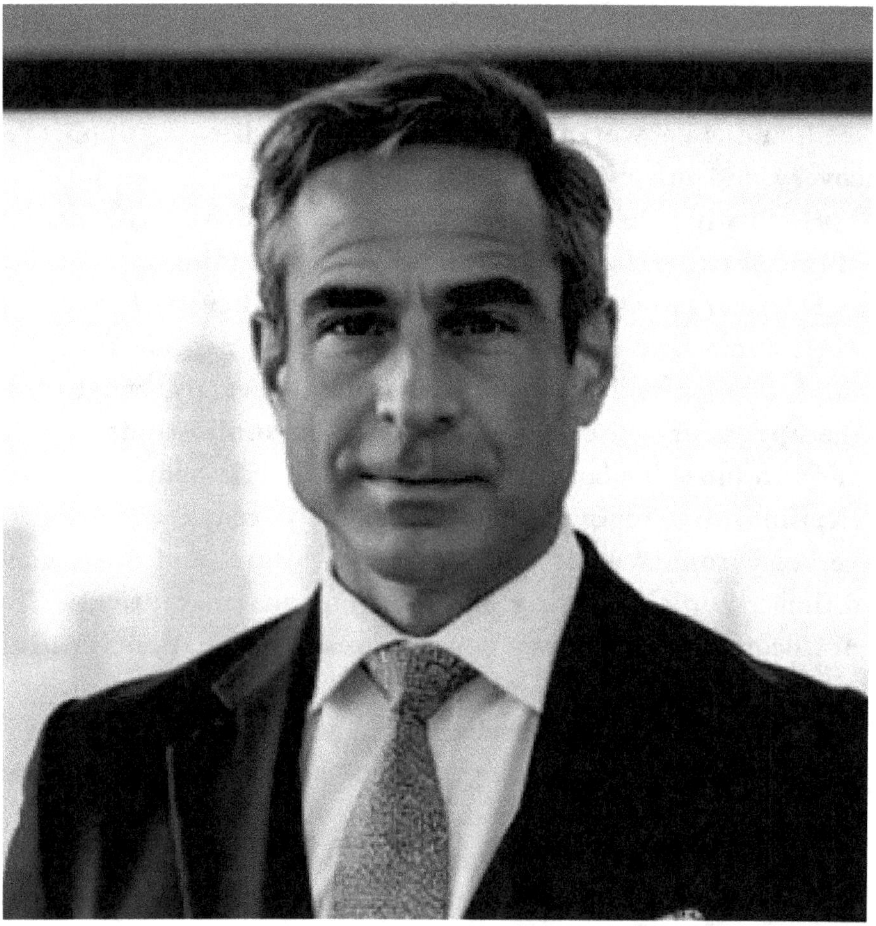

Dr. George Yiachos is a board-certified cardiologist and nuclear cardiologist, who also holds certifications in functional medicine, peptide therapy, and bioidentical hormone replacement therapy (BHRT). He is a fellow of the American Association of Ozonotherapy, the cardiology panelist for the BHRT Academy,and sits on the Medical Advisory Board for the Ozone Training Academy. He is a trailblazer in cutting-edge therapies designed to optimize health and vitality.

Driven by a deep commitment to achieving the best outcomes for his patients, Dr. George has embraced integrative medicine as a powerful approach to prevent disease, support recovery, and enhance overall well-being.

He firmly believes in prioritizing Health Span—the quality of life we experience—over merely extending life.

Dr. George has become expert in ozonotherapy (including MAH Ozone and EBOO), Prolozone therapy, peptide formulations, bioidentical hormone replacement therapy, weight loss therapy, neural therapy and innovative applications of PRF and exosomes for both sexual health and orthopedic recovery. His innovative regimens have successfully treated and even reversed coronary artery disease, heart failure, and other conditions, while reducing reliance on pharmaceuticals. His protocols have also shown powerful results for patients dealing with long-haul COVID and post- COVID vaccine complications.

In 2021, Dr. George founded WPR Heart and Health, a multistate integrative cardiology practice specializing in cellular medicine and regenerative therapies, with locations in Naples, Florida, and Long Island, New York.

His mission is to educate and empower patients to harness their body's natural ability to heal through nutrition, healthful lifestyle, and advanced integrative therapies.

https://WPRMedical.com

Heart Of The Matter

Heart Of The Matter

Dr. George Yiachos

License

www.ingramcontent.com/pod-product-compliance
Lightning Source LLC
LaVergne TN
LVHW022212200926
848481LV00006B/1938